The choice is yours and always has been

PSYCHOLOGY OF WEIGHT LOSS

Results in 21 days

Wayne Lambert

PSYCHOLOGY OF WEIGHT LOSS

Wayne Lambert

PSYCHOLOGY OF WEIGHT LOSS

By Wayne Lambert – ACSM, HFS - Health and Fitness Specialist

Master Neurolinguistic Practitioner and Nutrition Specialist

CEO of Wellness Fitcoach and Weight Loss Dubai

Founder of www.wellnessfitcoach.com

Author of 'Why Not Stay Fat? Maximise your fitness potential and Exercise Therapy - rehab exercises'

Important

I dedicate this book to my late grandparents,

Kind and gentle individuals with compassionate souls, who inspired me more than they could ever have imagined. I know they are all watching over me.

This book is also dedicated to your permanent weight loss success.

May 'Psychology of Weight Loss' provide you with everything you desire.

"It's now time to stop wishing your life away, make your dreams a reality!"

- Wellness FitCoach

ACKNOWLEDGEMENTS

As always, I need to thank my wife Laila, who continues to inspire me on a daily basis. I thank her wholeheartedly for her unconditional support in everything I do. I would also like to thank my daughter Eden Star, who keeps me grounded and teaches me that if you have the love and support of your family and friends, then in reality nothing else really matters.

FOREWORD

I have known Wayne for over 20 years now. When I first met Wayne I quickly learnt he is a determined spirit and dedicated beyond belief to his commitments and interests. I guess his career choice of entering the forces was an obvious career path to utilise this determination and dedication. As Wayne's career grew so did his hunger for explanations and understanding of his interest and beliefs regarding weight loss, health and fitness, and all round well-being. I would often see Wayne studying, researching, wanting more answers and listening to people and their experiences. The passion for the truth and explanations just grew within Wayne and the more he found out, the more areas deeper and wider he explored. A dedication to this day I still find extremely admirable and inspiring. Wayne as he always did, never minded people asking questions
and sharing his knowledge.

A few years ago I personally became in need of some advice. As a woman I had experienced the yo-yo diets and fads that come in and out of season. Chance made me meet Wayne again and before I knew it he was asking me to consider the whole package – total physiological thought process that embedded body and mind to a healthy combined package. His knowledge, explanations and unbiased straight talking, immediately hit home. I found myself answering my own questions too and facing reality. This was humbling and the first time I had realised the physiological impact and presence of my thoughts.

Knowledge is powerful if used appropriately, and suddenly I had cold hard facts staring at me. This made sense at last. Wayne never preached to me and didn't try to hard sell me with the miracle answer – his approach was to give me the answers and help me piece this crazy jigsaw of mind and body together. I remain today happier and healthier because of this and still inspired by Wayne's dedication and hunger for logical and lateral thinking. I have since specialised within teaching and truly believe the seed for being able to share something I know from the core originally came from the person I admire and have utmost respect for – Wayne Lambert.

• Barbara Ann Barter Hons HSC

TABLE OF CONTENTS

INTRODUCTION

"A march of a thousand kilometers begins with a single step."

- Chairman Mao

The aim of writing this book is to supply you with all the information you need to know about how you can lose weight and keep it off for the rest of your life. The content within this book has been collated from many years of health, fitness and lifestyle coaching; helping normal people like you achieve what you desire the most. Getting you to the weight management phase is our goal for you. Therefore, this book is strategically designed so that together we can produce a life-long program for you, not everyone reading…just you.

You may have all the reasons in the world to change something about yourself but inevitably never seem to get round to it. Therefore, you are consistently almost getting in shape. Psychology of weight loss can help you to overcome many mental obstacles that are keeping you overweight. For a number of reasons you may have spent your life getting on and off the weight loss merry-go-round, wasting time, starting, stopping, and maybe even lying about your behaviour i.e. making lame excuses and forever waiting for that right time to start (which incidentally never really comes), getting frustrated, complaining about genetics and generally being miserable.

Creating physiological change to get smaller, fitter, lighter or leaner seems to be more about the head than it is about the body. The weight loss process isn't as much about dumbbells, treadmills and carbohydrates as it is about attitude, thinking, beliefs, passion, self-control, decisions, standards and habits. Everyday people want everyday solutions. Psychology of weight loss is extremely important because it provides you with a foundation from which you can work from, incorporating the body and mind together.

In order to lose weight you must have support. So from this moment on, and as of today we want to offer you ours. We hope that this book will get you to where you want to be, but by giving you a lifetime of continuous support we believe that this in itself is priceless and we can continue to support you whenever you require it. Our offer of support is for your reassurance so that you know we are here for you every step of the way on your journey to permanent weight loss success. This book includes specialist advice on nutrition and physical activity, and in order for you to succeed on your journey to permanent weight loss you must learn how to make your mind and body work for you. It is extremely important that you understand what you are about to embark upon; it is a journey that you should not be turning back from, no more past struggles, only future intentions and justified decisions.

1

Why should you work with me?

This book has been written by myself, a former Royal Marine Commando, Physical Training and Rehabilitation Specialist, and I have been doing this and many other things since 1996. I have worked in many parts of the world and helped many people achieve their goals, but one thing is for certain and the most important thing I have learnt, is that if you want to continue dreaming, this is not the book for you. However, if you want to get out of your comfort zone and get results, then I am here for you.

I have four jobs at present: 1) I advise the military on all aspects of physical training and rehabilitation. 2) I tutor assess and internally verify health and fitness courses for some of the most renowned international awarding bodies. 3) I have my own personal training clients that I give 110% of my time to, before, during and after I train them. 4) I have my own Wellness FitCoach business that works alongside this book and my other projects such as personal development, business coaching and hosting courses.

But one thing is certain…I get results. So I hope this proves to you that I don't mess about, I also do these projects because I want to assist the global health initiative in order to help the millions of people in the world do something about their health. This life is a great journey and if we allow it, we can live longer by doing some really simple things. But if we don't help ourselves, then our bodies will just give up on us irrespective of how awesome the human body is.

WARNING
If you're reading this book searching for some kind of sympathy, then you have found the right book. We can sympathise because the greed of each nation has led you down a path of self-destruction. If you get easily offended or you get hurt by hearing truthful remarks about your weight, then you should read on because there is only compassion within this book. However, if you're not willing to get off your backside and move each and every day then you might as well go and get back in bed or lounge around on your sofa and fester.

If however, you want to lose weight permanently and live a fantastically happy life full of energy and hope then it will definitely be beneficial for you to read on.

How is this book different?

- We try to steer clear of the past i.e. our aim is not to dwell on past weight loss attempts, and the reasons why diets don't work
- We assume you probably know how and why you are where you are today, we also assume that you know more than you think about what you need to do to lose weight; we just nudge you in the right direction

- Our aim is to move you forward and get you to relate more positively to life; this book will endeavour to erase your past attempts and help to reset your mind
- It doesn't get you to count calories as such, just tells you what to try and change if you can
- I have tried to keep it as simple a procedure as possible for you, and for that reason kept all scientific jargon to a minimum. However, all reference materials used in this book and resources accessed are written at the rear of the book should you require it.

Wellness FitCoach's promise

Your route to achieving whatever you desire related to health and fitness will be as easy and progressive as you choose. Together (you and I) we won't be taking any shortcuts, but it will be a new lifelong journey for us.

To get the most out of this book I suggest you:
1. Read the book from start to finish
2. Complete each task
3. Start and complete 21 days in a row, utilising *everything* you have learned in this book.

If implemented and acted upon correctly, 21-days is the amount of time it takes to ensure your new overhaul becomes habitual for permanent weight loss success for the rest of your life. Among many things, this book can help you understand your mindset and assist you in obtaining control of your weight for long-term permanent weight loss success.

Actions
For this book to work for you, we suggest that you follow our instructions and you must stop what you are doing and take action wherever you see this symbol:

♥ Task

♥ = Our way of saying implement what we are asking of you and start to love and respect yourself once and for all. Your body is a highly intelligent machine but machines break, so we must assist where we can in order for it to function the best it can.

💡 = Whenever you see this symbol, a handy idea is suggested that you may find helpful on your weight loss journey.

Our task

Our task within this book is to take you from 'not knowing enough about how to lose weight' towards 'having the skills to lose weight without actually thinking about it.' Having belief in the ability you currently have is one thing, but the belief we want you to have once you have read this book will ensure you have all the resources you need for permanent weight loss success so long as you do the following:

- Complete all the tasks
- Use your self-talk dialogue effectively every moment that it's required
- Make the appropriate 'mind/body' habitual changes
- Ensure your daily choices (thoughts/nutrition/physical activity) are in line with your goals
- Continue to take action and behave according to your values, beliefs and desires.

Remain in a resourceful state

All that is required from you in order to get what you want is *flexibility* and a *willingness to experiment* to learn new skills. The more flexible you are with your thinking and behaviour the more successful you will be at getting the outcomes you want. You now know how important your unconscious mind is, so what is required of you now is to learn to communicate with it so that you can harness your resources. (Boyes, C., 2006.)

"The only way to keep your health is to eat what you don't want, drink what you don't like, and do what you'd rather not."

- Mark Twain

Part 1: ACCOUNTABILITY

Welcome aboard!

The following quote I believe is what permanent weight loss success is all about:

"Motivation is the art of getting people to do what you want them to do because they want to do it."

- Dwight D Eisenhower

♥Task 1
Sign on the dotted line that you agree to follow the guidelines in this book.

I …………………….agree that in order to lose weight successfully, I must do all the tasks and implement all the strategies in this book for 21 days (non-stop).

Signature: …………………..

NOTE
Unfortunately stress, anxiety and addiction can all limit the conscious control you have over your choices, which all affect the control you have.

Wellness FitCoach basic guidelines

Mind
Always remember that however difficult your past was doesn't need to determine your future self – sometimes however you may need to seek professional advice. Think positive thoughts about everything, and have no excuses at all for not knuckling down with your tasks and process goals. Deal with all negative past influences prior to beginning your 21-day challenge.

Nutrition
You wouldn't put something other than petrol or diesel in your car would you? So before you consume something (food and drink wise) look at it first and if you can recognise what it is and you can account for every single ingredient within its recipe then go ahead fuel yourself. However if you cannot then you could be setting yourself up for self-poisoning. Regarding fast 'junk' food, think about whether the meat is real and not processed, the hidden calories in ketchup, mayo and dips, not forgetting the amount of sugar that's in fizzy drinks, etc. I was always taught to drop a coin into the bottom of a glass of a fizzy drink and that put me off for life. Think natural as much as you can, or even better home grown i.e. no chemicals, preservatives just plain old fresh food. Learn to say NO to questions like, 'would you like fries with that' or 'would you like to upsize' or 'would you like cream on your mocha', etc.

5

Physical activity

If you decide to start by walking, walk with intention i.e. not as if you are on the promenade, so walk as if you are late for an important appointment. If you are starting out with exercise always do what you are capable of doing and try to maintain or progress from what you did in the last session. Always plan what you are going to do, this way you are halfway there, keep a diary or log your achievements so you can refer back to what you have already done. Exercising in the morning is better for most people because this way you are halfway through the session before you're awake and more importantly you enjoy it once you get going and you'll definitely feel fantastic afterwards. If you plan for a later workout you have the rest of the day to talk yourself out of it. *Number 1 rule = failing to plan is planning to fail*, so plan to have no excuses for exercise unless you're sick or injured and even then you can do alternative exercises working around the injury itself.

Summary of all
- *Thinking* about changing something about your thoughts, nutrition and exercise is good, so long as it's positive and it assists you with your requirements
- *Doing* something that assists you with your requirements is even better
- *Continuing to do something* until you have what you want is living the dream.

Wellness FitCoach ideology

Where there's a will, there's a way!

First, we must rid you of any excuses you may have, and you may have all the excuses under the sun as to why you are overweight, but know this...
I will find a way to counteract 99.9% of any excuses you may have.

This is the way I see it:
1. You need help
2. I have the tools and experience to help you
3. Together we will get there.

Excuses are barriers and one way or another barriers that are built can be overcome.

What's your excuse?

- It's in your genes...well, it doesn't have to be, so change the way you function and the way your children live; this book will help you do that
- I don't eat that much...well, that is a possibility, but so is self-denial, but let's address that later
- I do enough exercise...well, that is also a possibility, but is it the right kind and do you challenge your body in the right way?
- I don't have time...well, you have to make time if you want to succeed, we will address your day-to-day planning and time management later.

<u>Focus on choice</u>
You have the following choices:
- To slow down your thought processes and regain control of your life
- To make the right choices in your life
- If you watch TV do it before, during or after you have exercised.

<u>Planning and recording</u>
The best thing you can do if you are planning on starting this plan in the new year is ask friends, family, etc. to buy you the following as Christmas gifts. If you are due to start at another time of the year ask for them for your birthday, Easter or simply as a gift to support you on this, your most important decision so far.
Go and get your Christmas, Easter or birthday presents booked!

♥Task 2
You need a diary to record all your efforts. Either way set aside some time and money for the following:
1. A large A4 pad of paper, which will become your new lifestyle diary, and also buy something to write with
2. A full set of exercise clothes (for all weathers). For example, shorts and t-shirt for indoors and waterproof tracksuit, hat if raining, sunglasses if sunny – obviously training shoes too (for running and for working out) perhaps cross trainers
3. Perhaps an iPod (or similar) for motivational purposes.

The Wellness FitCoach treatment plan

<u>Choose the right time for you to get started</u>
So many people that want success are waiting for that perfect moment in order to start doing something about their current state. Unfortunately that perfect moment never arrives, so what are you waiting for? Change is always happening for the good of you and for everyone around you. It is the evolution of life. Is this your time to change?

<u>Do what you need to do – today</u>
Take action now and do the things that you want to do, with no excuses. You may have heard of the saying, "Don't put off until tomorrow what you can achieve today", well this is so important because if you don't start then how are you ever supposed to succeed?

♥Task 3
When are you going to start? Decide on a day/date/time/place when you will begin the 1st day of the rest of your life, (write it down, record it as an official appointment – *make yourself accountable*).

Treat the build-up to this moment as the most important priority you have ever had. More important than a job interview for a job you desperately need in order to put food on the table. For example, I will start as soon as I have read this book and as soon as I have taken action with all the tasks, because I am so sick and tired of waiting and trying the latest diet craze that doesn't really work for me. This book is about me and how I can help myself, using my own willpower and a newly learnt strategy of self-discipline and time management.

IMPORTANT
When you think about starting, remember that you are about to refresh your mind and body (physical activity-wise and nutritionally). It's not going to be painful, but it has to get you out of your comfort zone in order to be successful.

"Permanent weight loss success does not take place in your comfort zone, the answer to your dreams happens outside of it."

- www.wellnessfitcoach.com

How much do you value your health?

♥Task 4
Let's assume that weight loss is your main outcome goal (if not, edit the words accordingly) so in order to find out your current values related to losing weight you must answer the following questions:
1. What is most important to you about losing weight?
2. How will you know when you have reached your weight loss goal?
3. What is the next most important thing about losing weight?
4. What else is important to you about losing weight?

Let's use health as an example
Q. Can you do without it?
A. You definitely wouldn't want to.
So, using the word 'health' is always a good way to start a weight loss programme due to the fact that when you make healthy changes you will lose weight along the way.

"If you keep doing what you have always done, you will always get the same results. If you change what you do, the reaction of people around you will change and your own response will be different."

- Carolyn Boyes

8

Do you actually want to do this?

Even if you are certain you can do a certain task, achieve a certain process goal and even think you can control the overall outcome goal, you should still ask yourself whether or not you actually want to *engage* in it or not. So even if you feel that you want to commit all your time and energy into this project, you should still plan your strategy carefully i.e. whether it's the project as a whole, each individual task, even down to the process goals. That's not negativity or doubt, it's a realisation that you have to be 100% set before you commit i.e. you have set aside 21 days (non-stop) and you are ready to go before day 1 commences.

♥Task 5
Ask yourself and write down 'what losing __kg/lb would do to your life, or what would it bring/mean to you personally?' Only then can your dream start to become a reality.

Some simple rules before you begin:
- Make your new vision (internal picture) bigger, more clear, add colour to it
- Get rid of 'so called' friends or people in your life who actually want you to be miserable, who like you the way you are, and who will perhaps not like you the way you want to be
- Slow your eating speed down to 25% speed, and then when full 'stop', chew and enjoy
- Be consciously aware of what you are doing with no distractions
- Eat when (truly) hungry again…and do not eat emotionally
- With exercise adherence create a belief system via a conviction to succeed
- Turn your thoughts from 'a stubborn impossible' to a 'definite maybe.'

"In order to achieve permanent weight loss success you must participate and cooperate in a process that will meet your positive intention."

- Wellness FitCoach

What have you decided about your destiny?

From this moment on, begin preparing for change by starting to think positively. Begin to really feel your thoughts and relate to them more visually too. Picture yourself already having what you want, looking the way you want to look, feeling the way you want to feel.

"The only person you are DESTINED to become is the person you DECIDE to be."

- Ralph Waldo Emerson

9

Ask yourself why? Why today? What makes today different to your other days of wanting to lose weight? i.e. Have you had a health scare? Is a member of your family pressurising you to lose weight? Write your reasons down.

IMPORTANT
The decision to lose weight has to be your decision and no one else's. Do it for you!

With any type of desire, especially weight loss, most people start out with great intentions and belief about *what* they want, *why* they want it and some people have even planned out *how* they're going to get what they want. What the majority of people fail to do though, is reset their mindset through powerful intention. You must want it bad enough for it to happen. It's as simple as that. So, if you really want to lose weight and
get in shape, *nothing* will stop you, so long as you are willing to do what it takes.

Imagine for a moment what things will be like if you don't do what you have planned? And if you don't get what you want? Write down how you will feel. The consequences are far worse if you don't achieve your goals, as you will be more stressed and disappointed in yourself.

Your motivational support

You must support yourself with a motivating strategy and try to adjust your default settings for long-term success.

Success strategies to achieve your goals
Julian Rotter, a clinical psychologist, claimed that people who have internal locus of control tend to work harder, for they believe that it's themselves who would create their own destiny. On the other hand, people with external locus of control do not work hard to improve. Research suggested that males have more internal locus of control than women; and so do older people and people belonging to higher professional posts.
Though it seems that the internal locus of control is much more desirable and is more successful, often it leads to terrible anxiety and even depression.

In the worst situations, people may start to think that they are incompetent. On the contrary, often people with external locus of control seem very relaxed, calm, and even happy. These people take life as it comes and at times they feel lucky, and at times unlucky, but they accept whatever they get. In order for success to take place your behaviours must go through some form of change, and this change must be positive and long-term i.e. permanent.

♥ Dream
♥ Believe
♥ Achieve

The more reasons you have for wanting to achieve your goals the more determined you will become so lets get started.

Be open to changes
As human beings are creatures of habit, most of us do not want to accept change and we try to avoid changes in our lives as much as possible. To cite an example, if the role of an individual at work changes, he might be hesitant to accept that initially, though it might be a positive move. It has been proven that even though people do better with change, they are somehow not willing to accept it.

The same holds true for our eating habits as well. If you ask anyone to go on a diet, they will be able to do so because they are aware that most dietary measures are only temporary, and they would surely be able to revert back after a certain amount of time. Also, if you ask people to undergo a change in their eating habits, they will be more than likely reluctant to do so. So in such cases, we must opt for small changes in habits but on a more regular basis, and this method ensures permanent weight loss success.

Life is simple
Are you happy? Yes = Keep going. No = Change something!

♥ Task 7
Make a note of the reasons why you want to lose weight. Find about 10 good reasons why you no longer want to be overweight. Then you can focus on why you want to reach your target and visualise how good life will be when you have achieved your desires, how you will look when that moment arises and, of course, how you will feel.

1. I want to lose weight..
2. I want to lose weight..
3. I want to lose weight..
4. I want to lose weight..
5. I want to lose weight..
6. I want to lose weight..
7. I want to lose weight..
8. I want to lose weight..
9. I want to lose weight..
10. I want to lose weight..

Use words like 'because I want', 'in order to' and 'so I can' but do not continue until you have written down your reasons, or cut them out to keep safe. Trust me when I say that you are already on your way to success, you just have to have faith.

Example, "I want to lose weight so I can walk on the beach and feel comfortable without people staring at me."

Obesity is a medical condition; therefore, you need a 'lifestyle change' type treatment in order for you to get better. There must be no magic pills allowed from this point on. As you are aware there are no pills that work for long-term weight loss success, but what if there were some? It would only give people licence to continue killing themselves anyway. Foods that are rich in nutrients, vitamins and fibre will become your new natural remedy.

What doesn't help?
- Fast lifestyles/fast food/fast excuses/fast weight gain
- TV (and the 1000s of food adverts).

Strength in numbers
Working on something so important to you can be very difficult and daunting on your own; therefore, we suggest to do the following:

♥Task 8
Make a list of ways in which you feel you can get support. For example:
- From a health professional like your doctor, a dietician, or a nutritionist
- Join a group specifically for weight loss or a gym with a personal trainer
- Locate a reputable Cognitive Behavioural Therapist or Life Coach
- Self-hypnosis
- Family and friends who genuinely want to help and support you.

Visit your health professional and write (♥take your diary) the following statistics:
- A full health check for free if possible (BP, HR, etc.)
- An updated BMI reading
- As many measurements of your body as you can such as your waist, hip, biceps, chest, thighs, etc.

Even though healthwise you should feel better on a daily basis, when you have measurements you can use them as a start point and then check them every 4-6 weeks and see your improvements.

The A-B-C

Chances are that you are in need of the following:
- Altering your **Attitude**
- Changing your **Behaviour**

12

- Reinstating <u>Control</u> of your life.

So through careful 'strategic' planning you need to do the following:
- Establish an <u>Attitude</u> of self-efficacy, a firm belief in your ability for each of your new tasks, and each situation that you face from now on
- Establish how any <u>Behaviours</u> of unhealthy eating, or an inactive lifestyle may have developed
- Establish a healthy lifestyle with confidence and self-<u>Control</u> around food and physical activity.

"What happens when you face your fear?"

- Brian Tracy

Fear of success or fear of failure?

Are you the kind of person who manages to bypass the actual challenge or the ordeal with the fear of failure? As this is not only pessimistic, it is also escapist in a way. The other obstacle is your surroundings and the people you interact with. Society imposes certain norms upon us in terms of what we eat, how we dress, etc. If these impositions are accepted, then how are we supposed to make headway? It will be very difficult to ever change anything.

Fear is one of the main factors that can prevent change of any kind, and not just the fear of change itself, but also the fear of failing to bring about that change. For example, being afraid of letting go of a way of life you are accustomed to. Are you apprehensive about whether you will be able to successfully switch to a new pattern of life? This kind of fear is embedded into some people right from childhood onwards, and these deep-rooted fears seriously damage your potential to bring about change.

Obstacles:
- Fear of failure
- Surroundings and negative people.

Do you have a fear of failure?

♥Task 9
Rid yourself of fear and doubt and from this moment on, think positively about your future; think at all times that you will get what you want, as long as you want it enough. Write down all the things you want related to your health. For example, I want to be able to walk without getting out of breath, I want to play with my children, etc.

13

Challenge *strategies* against *fear*

Use 'challenges' such as poor health, a life threatening disease, etc. for a good purpose to strengthen yourself and others. Gain strength from your misfortune. For example, if you have had a health scare then you should automatically 'value' your life more; at least more than you did.

Reset your default

How competitive are you, and are you ready for the Wellness FitCoach challenge?
Some people say that they are not competitive. My belief however is that we are, even if it's with ourselves. In one way or another I believe that our nature is to be better than other people, whether it is at playing football or looking better than the next person when you go out to a bar or disco, etc. With weight loss my belief is that when you treat it like an event you can create better results for yourself by simply wanting to lose more weight, or even looking or feeling better than someone else whose desires are the same.

Being in a support group with like-minded people can assist with your competitiveness, but in reality it should start from within; wanting to be better than you were or are now. Your inner competition should be to delete your past and aim to be better tomorrow than you are today.

Begin to create the results that you desire; create a new attitude for success as if you have just been reborn and given a second chance. Start to invest in your health, and weight loss and many more benefits will follow with great speed; this is pretty much GUARANTEED.

Unlock your full potential
Believe it or not you already possess the tools you need to succeed, you just need the key in order to access your own resources.
"The choices you make now, the people you surround yourself with, they all have the potential to affect your life, even who you are, forever."

- Sarah Dessen

Regrets

Wellness FitCoach has an important rule about regrets. **Do not have any!**

Task checklist

Part 1: Accountability

☐ ♥ Task 1

Sign on the dotted line that you agree to follow the guidelines in this book.

☐ ♥ Task 2

You need a diary to record all your efforts.

☐ ♥ Task 3

When are you going to start?

☐ ♥ Task 4

Current values related to losing weight questions.

☐ ♥ Task 5

Ask yourself and write down 'what losing __ kg/lb would do to your life, or what would it bring/mean to you personally?' Only then can your dream start to become a reality.

☐ ♥ Task 6

Ask yourself why? Why today?

☐ ♥ Task 7

Make a note of the reasons why you want to lose weight.

☐ ♥ Task 8

Make a list of ways in which you feel you can get support.

☐ ♥ Task 9

Rid yourself of fear and doubt and from this moment on.

Part 2: PSYCHOLOGY

Life is a continuous journey of development and adjustment but the idea of change frightens some people. So when you learn to focus on valuing yourself, other people and the situations you face, then this will almost certainly lead you to greater happiness and a better quality of life. Change is not a threat and you are never too old to change, you also possess the right skills to make as many changes as you need in your life.

Psychology is the science of the mind and behaviour, the first part of the word 'psychology' comes from the Greek word psyche meaning *breath, spirit, soul*. Whichever way you choose to think, whether it's through meditation, religion or universally, your thoughts will always influence how you feel, and this in itself determines whether you enjoy life or not. The saying 'life is too short' is a good place to start, and as soon as you learn to enjoy each and every moment and be more appreciative of what you have, only then can you become your own master. People go through life chasing everything in the material world however, the greatest treasure of all is within you.

Positive psychology
Success is aided by a balance towards optimism, according to the psychologist Dr Martin Seligman who has researched optimism extensively. His research demonstrates that being optimistic increases your health, longevity, your morale and motivation amongst many other things. Being more positive gives you hope and energises you to action, and this will give you belief that you can be successful, which is more likely to make you so.

Root causes

There is definitely no rush with this phase and you need to get this part right for the remainder of the book to work.
You must address any underlying issues in order for weight loss to be successful and permanent. If you don't do this you will always be returning back to this starting point.

♥Task 10
Address your lifestyle patterns as follows:
*   From waking up in the morning until you go to bed
*   Write down everything that you do – absolutely everything
*   You need it to be like a food diary, a physical activity log, and a how you're feeling throughout the day-type diary.

Writing things down will make you more aware of what your day really entails as opposed to what you think it entails. For example, if you suddenly feel low in energy then recall what you last had to drink or eat, this could be your answer.

"When you finally let go of the past something better always comes along."

- Anon

For example, weight gain can be used as a form of protection from the root cause. What's your root cause to poor health? More specifically, *find out the root cause for your weight gain.*

♥Task 11
- • Work out what it is that's bothering you
- • Pinpoint the thought
- • Explain the thought fully and then summarise (♥write in your diary) the most upsetting part about it
- • Question it. Is it the real reason?
- • Expand your thinking (repeat).

Repeat this process, but be flexible and creative.

"As you grow older, you'll find the only things you regret are the things you didn't do."

- Zachary Scott

WARNING
If you cannot get to the root cause of your weight gain then you definitely may need to seek professional assistance from a cognitive behavioural therapist for example.

This book wants you to relate to always getting what you want, and even though we don't preach religion or a higher being, we would still like you to believe in your faith to attract exactly what it is you want. We don't really quote the law of attraction either, but this is a belief that the universe mirrors back to you exactly what you are holding inside of you i.e. if you look at yourself and feel dissatisfaction you will continue to attract feelings of dissatisfaction. Try and manipulate your feelings and you will see for yourself. Turn negative thoughts of not having what you want into positive thoughts and feelings as if you already have what you want and as the law suggests, the same attraction exists within you i.e. 'whatever you want' – 'you can attract' – 'therefore you can have'.

Psychological & emotional reasons

Body image psychology study
Feelings and emotions keep changing continuously according to our external and internal surroundings, but in the long run this also affects our perceptive capabilities. Your body image, which is sensitive to moods, emotions and the retention of water, and more importantly weight, is therefore characterised by a complex blend of its physical and psychological aspects. In 2000, a body image psychology study was carried out by the Psychiatric department of University of British Columbia. They published a comparative study of 21 normal women and 21 women suffering from anorexic nervosa. And the study proved that the anorexic women were prone to suppressing anger and negative feelings to a great extent. The convoluted psychological issues, which lead to a poor body image, do not always end up as eating disorders; however, they are capable of causing severe damage to your body and mind. You must know that bulimia or anorexia is not caused by poor body image alone, as this can happen to anybody and everybody, and it is also capable of affecting school goers and teenagers.

Another comparative study was carried out by the University of Melbourne (School of Psychology) in Australia for a period of 16 months. The School of Psychology evaluated the importance of biological, psychological and social models when it comes to clarifying body image among both normal and overweight boys and girls. The analysis showed that the group of overweight kids mostly suffered from low self-esteem as they strived to lose weight. This was brought about by the unhealthy comparison between the overweight and their peers whose weights were within a normal range.

A 12-month study by the University of Washington took matters a step further. The researchers carried out the study based on the experiences of Grade 7 and Grade 10 girls and boys, and the study showed that body dissatisfaction and psychological factors that naturally followed it up often influenced social and peer relations. While boys were prone to comparing themselves with muscular idols of their dreams, dissatisfaction among girls was chiefly caused by appearance comparison, and conversations among friends and acquaintances. The study was published by the journal of Developmental Psychology in 2004.

Another study published in 2006 in the Journal of Clinical Child and Adolescent Psychology by the School of Psychological Science in Melbourne, traced how body dissatisfaction often led to extreme depression and low self-esteem. However, the time has come for people to realise that only carrying out body image psychology studies will not help in improving the social conditions and the health conditions of the individuals concerned. Time has come for us to move on from the why and how, and take adequate steps that will help people deal with their perceptions and cope with eating disorders. (Geller, Cockell, Hewitt, Goldner & Flett, 2000) (Carlson Jones, Vigfusdottir & Lee, 2004)
(Paxton, Neumark-Sztainer, Hannan & Eisenberg, 2006)

It is very difficult to control hunger and starve yourself; also getting back to normal eating has a yo-yo effect with your weight. The reasons why a person reaches obesity are quite vague, but there are books that say that obese people eat excessively out of habit, although this reference overlooks the psychological and emotional reasons. Counsellors who write on this subject concentrate on the psychological problem only.

Four situations that say that excess fat is due to some psychological disorder:
1. Think back in time when you were slim and had attained, even though not completely, your aim to lose excess weight. Think about whether or not you were extremely active then, or whether you were working out a lot. Depending on your answer then your fat may have had something to do with some mental discomfort.
2. In case, after the completion of your diet your weight increases by more than a pound of fat in one week, it is most likely that your excess weight, before your dietary measure, was due to some mental issue. Excluding the possibility of addictive allergy infections.
3. Bulimia and anorexia, the diseases associated with food problems, are in most cases due to some psychological problem.
4. Your weight could be due to improper mental composure, especially if your overeating is sparked off by stress and anxiety. You can take into account your mental and emotional difficulties in case you have started gaining weight during your teenage years. Probably they are the reasons why you cannot shed your excess fat now. In case your excess weight is due to some intense emotional shock that you have confronted in those years, then you will have a tough time trying to become thin today.

A very small number of fortunate people all over the world are successful in recognising the emotional problem that causes their obesity, and immediately transform the problems into ways of how to be slim. However, most people confront many difficulties and undertake rigorous practices to become thin. They try all means possible; knowing very well that in spite of all their efforts their being gracefully slim is not a result they can be sure of. Quite a number of books define emotionally stressful situations that give rise to the binging habit.

Generally, it is the emotional upheavals as well as the various circumstances that we confront in life that increase our stress. Therefore, in order to escape from them a person might endeavour to eat too much, and if that makes that person comfortable, then they continue to overeat. At times, we run away from feelings such as love, annoyance, desire, and sorrow, etc. and tend to find an alternative in food.

We sometimes cannot come to terms with the idea that we are just another statistic, or just another one in the rat race. At times people have parents who keep feeding their children or parents rebuke them by telling them that they will not be allowed to eat, or any other such childhood shock related to food gives rise to this problem. We always tend to consciously ignore that aspect about ourselves, which leaves us

19

stressed and weary because the moment any incident reminds us of that shock we are left drained psychologically.

People who suffer from emotional distresses connected to food, then binge. The only remedy is to stay calm in such circumstances, but the person suffering from it will know that it is rather difficult. It requires a lot of willpower and inner strength to relax in such situations, and then gradually try and transform yourself into how you want to be.

Looking upon fat as a kind of sign such as fear, a pain in the head or even excess intake of alcohol helps to combat the problem. The emotional reasons that lead to these disorders are quite similar.

The upcoming chapters of this book will assist you immensely in case you have recognised that the causes for your excess weight are emotional.

Is it emotional?
It is essential that you accept the fact that food has the powers to help you cope through very difficult situations of stress; therefore, it is important that you understand that your body craves for food, not only when you need food but also when you need any emotional comfort. So it is vitalthat you learn how to segregate the call of your body for food, from the call of your body for food to get emotional satisfaction.

Your thought processes

Behaviour patterns and overeating
The diet patterns of humans have changed rapidly over the years and meals no longer consist of freshly made food high in nutritional value. The food no longer contains the essential carbohydrates, vitamins, minerals, water, unsaturated fat, micronutrients, etc. On the contrary, it consists of nicotine, caffeine, alcohol, preservatives, cholesterol, modified fats, starch, etc. This is mainly because of a culture of fast food and packaged foods, which are easy to cook.

Such a diet is not only unhealthy and leads to an immediate onset of obesity, but it also deprives the body of the essential nutrients that it needs. You must remember that your body remains unsaturated when it comes to these nutrients, and as a result tries to get them from the unhealthy food that you eat, which as a consequence has precious little to offer. This unfortunately results in gross overeating of unhealthy foods. The behavioural patterns of most people with respect to spending money are also strange. With people's incomes increasing, it has been observed that people don't use this money to buy healthy food. The quality of food that they themselves eat does not go up with a rise in income.

On the contrary, the nutrition content in their food that is important for a proper functioning of the body reduces with the increase in income! Huge national losses are also a major concern for the nation as a whole. A large number of workdays are lost because of some obesity related problem or another. Insurance claims are made frequently for such problems, and companies also spend more on their employees' health, consequently incurring large expenses.

Negativity

Express your feelings in suitable ways because bottling up negative feelings can be worse if these are creating physical ailments. It is perfectly fine to inform those close to you about your source for concern. Nevertheless, be aware that your loved ones may be powerless to properly support you in dealing with your feelings. When this occurs, take the advice and support of an outsider about the circumstances – like a counsellor, your family doctor, holistic therapist or even someone religious or spiritual to guide you with your emotional health. Live a balanced life and don't attempt to think about situations that raise negative feelings like troubles at home, work or school.

You do not have to act happy when you are emotionally unstable, but you can try and change your mindset to a positive one by being grateful for what you do have as opposed to what you do not. If you try to emphasise the good things in your life rather than dealing with depressing feelings, you can at least change the way you feel through positive thought processes.

You might want to keep a journal to record the things that make you smile and feel at peace. Your quality of life can be improved and your fitness can recover, as proved by studies. You have to search for ways to get rid of stressful and overpowering negative things in your life, so take out time for things you get pleasure from.

Calm your mind and body, as your emotions can be balanced through constructive methods of relaxation like meditation. It is a type of guiding thoughts, available in several manifestations. For instance, you may meditate through exercise, breathing deeply and stretching. You can take your holistic therapists or doctor's guidance on means of relaxation. Take care of your body to ensure excellent emotional health, this can be by a regular schedule of eating nutritious food, sleeping as much as necessary and exercising to mitigate hidden tension. At all costs you should aim to avoid overeating.

Can negative thoughts be keeping you fat?

Human beings nearly always lean towards negative or pessimistic thinking, and this has a profound effect on our psyche and lifestyle. Research has shown, from childhood onwards, an average person hears NO about 50,000 times and YES only 8,000 times. So negative thinking is very deeply ingrained in us. So if you think negatively, then in real life losing weight becomes almost impossible, and this kind of pessimistic thinking will gradually pervade your brain and from a conscious thought it sinks down to the level of the subconscious. It becomes a loop you cannot break out of.

Fact

Almost 96% of your behaviour is determined by your subconscious, these subconscious thoughts determine your day-to-day activities, and if these thoughts are negative then they will definitely prevent you from losing weight because they induce you to think you can never lose weight. Usually weight loss programs include a diet and a workout regimen, as these combined are very important; therefore, you must not ignore the mind-body connection. While dieting you are constantly affected about how terrible the diet is or while exercising you feel reluctant to perform the exercises, or you doubt their effectiveness. With this way of thinking you have no hope of losing much weight in the long-term.

It's very difficult in the beginning to actively love diet food, but the trick is to focus on something else and drive the negative thoughts away from your mind. Discipline your mind as well to think about things you actually like, as this is the only way to retain an optimistic frame of mind. Your mental activities have to correspond with healthy eating and exercise. You have to back it up with support from your mind and only then can you hope for success. The advantage here is that your mindset is something you *can* control and monitor. It's your choice, think about the wonderful things that accompany loss of weight, think about the positive side and do whatever it takes and make that choice.

Interrupting negative eating patterns

Weight loss hypnosis is one of the greatest tools for fighting negative eating patterns that plague our modern society. The reasons behind people developing these negative eating patterns are various and complex, but people need to be made aware of how their habits affect them and how they need to be changed.

How your mind is affected by food

The human mind is fragile. The entire system is interconnected through a mass of neurons, and this connection is so sensitive that if even one link of the entire chain is missing, the connection snaps and the mind goes wobbly. The mind is considered the strength of the human body. But at the same time it is extremely vulnerable to all kinds of attacks. A simple fever can make the mind go blank and during very high fever, several people say all sorts of things they have no recollection of when they are back to normal. This is because they have lost a hold on their minds. The mind, more so than the body, needs proper nutrition for its proper functioning. Food must be eaten not only for a healthy body, but also for a healthy and well-functioning mind. Caffeine, nicotine, chocolate overdose, etc. cause the mind even greater damage than they cause the body. Such food substances cause havoc in the entire neurological system. The neurotransmitters may get blocked because such foods are certainly not what they need; therefore, are not welcomed by them.

'Holistic' thinkers have existed for a long time, constantly repeating the philosophy that the body and the mind are inextricably interconnected, and that any tiny trouble in one affects the other. In the 70s and the 80s, science discovered a connection path called neurotransmitters and realised that the philosophy of those ancient thinkers was true. Scientists even now believe the thought that the mind and the body are linked in such inextricable terms that it is difficult to separate one's activities from another's.

Example
Here's where you can get a brief look into the neurotransmitter model that scientists came up with. First, to understand what these neurotransmitters actually do, they are responsible for maintenance of the alertness chemicals and the calming chemical. These two chemicals are absolutely indispensable in the human body and the human mind. They are responsible for the thought process to happen smoothly.

Now, the two main macronutrients in the body are proteins and carbohydrates. These nutrients transmit the neurotransmitters making it possible to generate the alertness and the calming chemicals in an effective manner, enabling the mind to be energetic and calm during times of stress. The nutrition intakes are all complementary to one another. The amino acids in protein foods are of various kinds. Now these vie for access to the brain and this helps create a balanced system within the body.

If you have attempted weight loss before, only for the same body fat to return, or if you have had the same health problems with the same negative results, then you may have been unconsciously running old negative programs in your head and re-enforcing them with negative thought patterns.

Some examples of negative thoughts are:
- I will never be able to lose this weight
- I won't be able to get into this exercise routine
- I can't control my eating
- It must be in my genes, so I give up.

Before you begin, you have to demolish, destroy and quite literally get rid of all past negative thoughts about weight loss, including everything you have told yourself in your head or have heard from others. Once these have gone from your mind and the record has been set straight, only then can you proceed further to replace those negative thoughts with positive ones and a realistic strategy for your successful, long-term weight loss journey.

♥Task 12
Lifestyle Challenge 1
In order to successfully change your attitude towards food and drink you must write down a minimum of 10 of your own phrases; phrases that you will need to repeat as

often as you can throughout the day and throughout the initial 21 days (non-stop). The results will be powerful, you'll see.

Some examples of positive self-talk phrases are:
- I promise myself not to eat fatty or sweet foods when I am tired or stressed
- I will have more energy when I cut my fat and sugar intake and increase exercise
- I will eat more high fiber and low-fat foods that I like
- I don't need to go on a starvation diet to lose weight
- I can handle stress without eating food, especially things I shouldn't be eating
- I am willing to try a healthy eating and exercise plan to lose and keep off excess fat
- I know how important water is, so I will drink more of it
- I will become leaner, healthier and happier after today.

Your very own positive self-talk phrases
1. I...
2. I...
3. I...
4. I...
5. I...
6. I...
7. I...
8. I...
9. I...
10. I...

Use powerful words such as 'I can', 'I will' and 'I am' unless of course, the sentence dictates otherwise. These phrases should go with you everywhere and try to place them wherever you can see them. These should be written down now or once you have read the relevant chapters, which will help you.

How can you improve your emotional health?
Try to identify your emotions and the causes behind their occurrence. You can manage your emotional health by identifying the grounds for stress, sadness and worry in your life.

If things really start to get on top of you and you feel yourself getting stressed, a good thing to try is an imagery exercise which is best explained by Helen Whitten (2009), who says that 'to take your attention away from your thinking you should focus on your heart area, to the core of your being, the solar plexus.' She mentions that this experience is a sensory one, an awareness of your 'presence' within the world, of how you're feeling physically and emotionally at that moment in time. The aim of the above exercise is to observe that your feelings should be observed

24

without judging yourself as good or bad, also to take you beyond thought. She suggests that you take a deep breath and imagine a feeling of balance spreading throughout your whole body so you feel peaceful, alive and alert.

You can build these types of mental images into any part of your future i.e. any situation or event you feel may benefit from such an exercise. Your aim at all times is for immersion to take place and for you to see yourself mentally present and balanced. Another useful exercise is to imagine that your body is exactly like a movie projector, and when you watch the film you see your life playing through the projector, depicting all your thoughts and feelings. Remember though that you have put everything into this film, so if there's a part of your film that you don't like then you just need to choose better thoughts and feelings to suit your needs. This can be done at any time because you have complete control of what goes into your film.

♥ Task 13

It is also important to understand the type of pattern that you associate with food. For example, you should maintain a food diary and write down all what you have eaten for a week. Make sure that you keep a note of what you felt after eating certain food types. Also write down what made you eat the food that you would not have otherwise eaten, after a week try and find a pattern in your food habits. You may find out that you eat the most when you are depressed or lonely. Maybe you eat most when you anticipate trouble at the work place, this way you can actually find out what your problem is and where it lies. You can also try and find alternative solution to your problem rather than binging on food. In case your career is what is causing you stress, you can take the help of a career counsellor. Or you can go out and join a club especially if you are feeling lonely.

Stress

Another factor that causes you to overeat is stress, as more than half of the people who are overweight admit that they overeat when they are stressed. They admit that in situations of stress, they eat unhealthy food. For example, they sway towards having a pizza, etc., whereas they could have easily consumed an organic smoothie or something as healthy.

Any stressful thoughts that you have lead to the release of cortisol, adrenaline, and nor-adrenaline in your body which suppresses your immune system. Too much stress in your life , excess sugar and stimulants are also likely to make matters worse. According to Kate Neil and Patrick Holford (1998) the net result of stress or a diet too high in sugar and refined carbohydrates is an inability to keep blood sugar levels stable. Raised insulin and cortisol increases your risk of inflammatory health problems too. They go on to say that the human race has now been subjected to countless man-made chemicals in our food and our environment. They recommend you to choose raw, organic foods as much as you can, and to make sure at least half your diet consists of raw fruit, vegetables, wholegrains, nuts and seeds.

25

Do you have a stressful life?

Stress is one of the most common killers of human beings. So from this moment on, promise yourself that you will take each moment, each second, every minute, hour and day in your stride, and live each breath as if it were your last. Write down ways in which you can reduce the stress in your life. For example, my boss works me into the ground but I must think about my family without a mother or a father if I carry on this path. Money is important but health and family is more so.

Emotional Freedom Technique (EFT)

Clearly, it is not possible or even recommended to eliminate stress entirely. However, you can work to provide your body with tools to compensate for the bioelectrical short-circuiting that can cause serious disruption in many of your body's important systems.

By using techniques such as the Emotional Freedom Technique (EFT), you can re-program your body's reactions to the unavoidable stressors of everyday life. Exercising regularly, getting enough sleep and meditation are also important 're-lease valves' that can help you manage your stress.

How does EFT work?
Working on its discovery statement that 'our negative emotions are caused by a disruption in the body's energy system', EFT works to clear such disruptions and eliminate the resulting emotional response or intensity to restore emotional harmony and offer relief from physical discomfort. This is done by focusing on the specific problem, whilst tapping with fingers on the end points of energy meridians. The combination of sending kinetic energy to our energy system whilst uncovering and focusing on root causes, facilitates a 'straightening out' of the energy system; thereby eliminating the 'short circuit' to the body's learnt response or negative emotion.

http://www.theenergytherapycentre.co.uk/eft-explained.htm

> *"Life is to be lived comfortably, not in a stressed out zone of worry or fear."*

> - Wellness FitCoach

Emotionally healthy people are already conscious of their behaviour, feelings and thoughts, and the stress and problems of their lives are negligible due to their knowledge of coping with them. They generally have fulfilling relationships and are more positive about themselves.

The things that can interrupt your emotional state and make you feel sad, anxious or stressed include:
• Losing your job

26

- A child leaving or returning home
- Coping with a loved one's demise
- Marrying or divorcing
- Enduring a disease or an injury
- Being promoted at work
- Undergoing financial troubles
- Shifting to a new house or giving birth.

Both 'good' and 'bad' changes can be equally stressful.

How can your emotions affect your health?
The frequently termed 'mind/body connection' is your body's response to your manner of thinking, feeling and acting. Your body attempts to inform you that things are unsuitable when you are worried or apprehensive. By way of an extreme example, a particularly stressful event like someone's death can lead to the growth of a stomach ulcer or high blood pressure.

The following physical signs indicate an imbalanced emotional health:
- Back ache
- Altered appetite
- Upper body pain
- Diarrhoea or constipation
- Dried up mouth
- Intense weariness
- Common aches
- Headaches
- High blood pressure
- Insomnia – sleeplessness
- Dizziness
- Palpitations – feeling hurried heartbeats
- Sexual troubles
- Shortness of breath
- Rigid neck
- Sweating
- Troubling stomach
- Change in weight.

Your body's immune system can deteriorate due to a poor emotional situation, making you susceptible to colds and other infections in emotionally turbulent times. At these times you will probably not take appropriate care of your health. You might not wish to exercise, eat nutritious food or take the doctors prescribed medicines. Another indication of poor emotional health is the abuse of tobacco, alcohol or other drugs.

Why does your doctor need to know about your emotions?

You may not be accustomed to discussing your feelings or personal problems with your doctor, but you must try and keep in mind that the doctor cannot possibly know you're stressed, disturbed or anxious just by seeing you. Be honest with him or her, especially if you note such emotions. The doctor will ensure that other health problems are not the cause of your physical symptoms. If other health problems are not the basis of the symptoms, then both you and your doctor can deal with the emotional reasons of these signs. The doctor's suggestions will treat your bodies warning signs, and thereafter both you and the doctor can tackle your emotional condition. If your intense negative feelings prevent you from enjoying life and do not disappear, then it is imperative for a medical consultation. These are the signs of 'major depression'. A medical disease treated with individualised counselling, holistic therapies or medicines, commonly referred to as depression.

When to see your doctor?

Do you feel that you have an eating disorder? Do you not feel full even after eating a sufficient quantity of food? Do you seem to eat a lot but despite that, you lose weight? Do you take laxatives or resort to vomiting to compensate for the extra calories that you have taken in? Are you always chronically depressed? If the answer to any of these questions is yes, then it is advisable that you must see a doctor at once. Most of the time we forget that sometimes we eat, not because of necessity but out of sheer habit. It does happen that no matter how full we are we still carry a bag of popcorn with us to the movie hall.

The same is the case when we are watching television at home, we do not open that bag of potato chips because we are hungry, we do so only because we are habituated to do so. People who eat in excess or have the dietary disorder bulimia, do not have any sense of control, they cannot help but eat a large quantity of food at a single sitting. People who are most prone to this disorder are the people who have tried their hand at dieting but have failed miserably; such people have very low self-esteem. There are many similarities between bulimia and anorexia, the most common being the cause.

Research

There seems to be a common occurrence of sexual and/or physical and emotional abuse in direct relation to both eating disorders (though not all people living with eating disorders are survivors of abuse). There also seems to be a direct connection in some people to clinical depression. The eating disorder sometimes causes the depression or the depression can lead to the eating disorder.

All in all, eating disorders are very complex emotional issues. Though they may seem to be nothing more than a dangerously obsessive weight concern on the surface, for most men and women suffering with an eating disorder there are deeper emotional conflicts to be resolved. Another class of people who are prone to eating disorder is the people who are addicted to a certain thing and are trying to quit.

For example, in case of chronic smokers who are trying to quit, there is a chance that they indulge in food, this is mainly because they need to keep their hands and mouth occupied. Most of the time, these people overcome the need for nicotine and replace it with the pleasure of food. According to many doctors, people who are prone to depression resort to food, and this gives them emotional support, which in turn helps them to forget about their depression for a while. It has been proven that in many cases it is not just the psychological factor that causes us to overeat; it is the brain that prompts us to indulge in overeating.

Cognitive Therapy

The prevalence of obesity has been on the increase and, on the whole, improvements in patient education have not led to the desired outcome of weight maintenance, let alone weight loss.

In more recent decades, behaviour modification approaches have also incorporated strategies from cognitive therapy, which have involved the identification and modification of 'dysfunctional' thinking patterns and consequent negative mood states, hence, the term 'Cognitive Behaviour Therapy' (CBT). There is increasing interest in adopting CBT approaches to achieve more modest and sustainable weight loss and improved psychological well-being. (K.L. Liao, 2000).

In this book you will learn specific techniques as part of your treatment plan, and when used correctly can give you long-term success.

This success can be achieved by using principles such as:
- Planning what you eat
- Scheduling your day to include food shopping and mealtimes
- Arranging your environment to support weight loss
- Planning for 'high-risk' situations such as a friend's birthday party
- Daily reading of written weight loss goal cards and dealing with counter-productive thoughts about food, such as 'I deserve this piece of cake' or 'I'll never lose the weight'.

In a Swedish study, the group randomised to receive Cognitive Therapy lost more weight and kept it off over the next 18 months, while those assigned to a waiting list gained weight over the same period. (Cognitive Therapy for Weight Loss developed by Judith Beck, Ph.D).

Cognitive psychology investigates internal mental processes, such as problem solving, memory, learning and language. So we have explained these below for you:
- *Solving the problem* of weight loss by utilising your mind and body (via thoughts and behaviours) building on your existing strengths
- *Testing your memory* by way of only using your past experiences if they are positive, also ensuring that you take all the correct tools and resources

29

with you into your newly formed habitual future that awaits you.
- *Learning* more about yourself through specific tasks, process goals and thought patterns i.e. self-talk
- *Language* – Selecting your terminology or dialogue for future success, and moving you away from talking about a problem towards talking positively and constructively about solutions. Your dialogue will relate to nutrition, physical activity and thinking before, during or after you act. We literally want you to talk to yourself (internally), so if you have behaved in a certain way we want you to ask yourself 'was that action congruent with my outcome goal?' And if yes, move onto the next process goal. If not then correct the thought and consequently correct your action with a new behaviour and learn from it. At all times replacing your language or dialogue with positivity and confidence, etc. Looking at the language of your body will allow you to have a more holistic approach related to your posture and how you carry yourself. Also being more confident by standing tall, being more assertive and having good interpersonal communication skills. Transforming your body language in addition to all the other approaches can assist you in having a more improved overall personal presence.

Cognitive theory is also what we encourage you to focus on, to focus extensively on your mental processes, so that once you have completed your tasks you take in the information through your senses and process the data mentally. The same goes for the process goals and even more so when you collate your self-talk dialogue.

However in depth you want to go with this project will dictate how successful you are, but the process is virtually the same, so that mentally you will automatically do the following:
- *Organise the data* – into a manageable and understandable language specific to you
- *Manipulate it* – fine-tune the content using methods that will work for you
- *Remember it* – with reminders on your phone, at your office desk, in your handbag, stored to memory
- *Relating it to information you had stored previously* – if you choose to use visualisation as one of your strategies for example, this could mean you having a clear picture in your head of how you would like to look, or a positive memory you have of how you were when you were younger, etc.

www.medicalnewstoday

Suggestion from Wellness FitCoach
Seek professional assistance from a cognitive behavioural therapist.
Or do it your way (DIY) ♥ *Pen and notebook required!*

Rational Emotive Behaviour Therapy (REBT)

A-B-C theory and loss of weight

Rational Emotive Behaviour Therapy (REBT) is one of the first behaviour therapies of a cognitive nature, which Albert Ellis came up with in 1953 in order to solve the specific problems of troubled individuals. Through REBT, which is largely based upon the A-B-C theory of personality, Ellis tried to propagate the idea that our emotions are entirely influenced by our beliefs, and not the events that we come across in our lives, as was commonly believed. Ellis was of the opinion that our emotional well-being and our beliefs are directly proportional.

It was his belief in his own theory, which ultimately became one of the most powerful in the hands of therapists looking to help their patients out by teaching them how to counter their irrational fears and replace them with rational beliefs. REBT suggests that the human mind has the capacity to think both rationally and irrationally. While rationality helps you to be objective in your approach, irrationality distorts, convolutes and misinterprets reality.

When it comes to the A-B-C theory mentioned above, **A** signifies some kind of an event that confronts you with a challenge you must pursue in your life. This is called an **activating** event, and an example of this might be that of a teenager being ditched by his lover. The **B** stands for the **belief,** which follows thereafter, affecting your individual emotions, which is in turn represented by the **C** – the **consequences** of how you feel and what you do. If you expect everybody to like you and treat you properly, then your behaviour can only be termed as irrational, as you are bound to feel let down because this can only lead to anger or depression. If, on the other hand, you are capable of behaving rationally, the disappointing and abrupt end to the relationship for example will not have a long-term effect on you.

IMPORTANT

The past is unchangeable and we must work upon replacing our irrational beliefs with rational ones instead in order to make our present much more pleasant. REBT has done a great deal to spread the word that psychological dysfunction is primarily caused by anxiety and depression, which are only parts of *human neuroses.* Irrational belief only convolutes your thought process and drives you deeper and deeper into the world of confusion and continuous self-negation as you set yourself unthinkable and almost impossible targets. You slowly develop a habit of continuously assessing them in a negative manner, while you juggle the 'should do', the 'ought to do' and the 'must do' unsuccessfully.

These self-effacing beliefs take root in your mind when you are just a child and then continue to grow as you keep revisiting them. This only proves that irrational beliefs can only result in unhealthy emotions, which at times tend to take a toll on you physically. According to the A-B-C theory, the consequences of possessing a negative mentality are generally mild, leading to procrastination on many occasions. But in certain scenarios, can also lead to dire circumstances, disrupting and immobilising your general well-being.

REBT, based largely upon the A-B-C theory, helps an individual suffering from self-effacing beliefs to overcome them and enjoy life on a larger and grander scale as they come to terms with their imperfections, which exist in all of us and are but only a part of life. A proper collaboration between the client and the counsellor treating them with REBT therefore, can only lead to positive results.

Be creative
Ignore at your peril the psychological skills of listening to your thoughts, and also listening to carefully selected music (music that you love to listen to) and watching personal motivational videos of perhaps others who have successfully lost weight to inspire you. This has been researched to enhance mental toughness.

Regarding music, there's a reason why you like a certain type of music. It puts you in a trance of where you prefer to be, or where you feel more comfortable and at ease. It has been suggested that music in particular, may elicit a number of psycho-physiological responses that lead to improved performance.

For example:
- By diverting the attention away from feelings of tiredness and fatigue
- By influencing states of arousal to either stimulate or calm the participant
- By making the activity seem easier through synchronisation and emulation of movement patterns to the music
- By decreasing negative mood and increasing positive mood.

Are your beliefs creating the change that you desire?

Because you have your own view on things, the way you think about something can be very different to somebody else's. Have in your mind though that your perception needs to be flexible as explained by Carolyn Boyes (2006), she suggests that your view *can be*, and in some cases *should be* changed in order to get different results.
Think about the following question: Is it possible that what you believe to be true about weight loss and how to lose weight may not be true?

♥Task 15
Attempt the following tasks to help you with the question:
- What is your overall perception about how you should think, act and behave in order to assist you to lose weight?
- What is your perception about nutrition, and what types of food and drink do you feel will assist you to lose weight?
- What is your perception about exercise, and what types of exercise do you feel will assist you to lose weight?

32

Carolyn Boyes gives the following advice:

- To make you more effective as a person you should always try to understand and respect that your beliefs and the way you value things may be different to other peoples
- The results you have had in your life so far may not be the results that you actually want, especially related to your health and weight, etc., but you need to understand that as humans we are extremely effective at getting results
- Your unconscious mind works perfectly, given the instructions it already has, and everything it does has positive intention.

She illustrates it best here by explaining in a step-by-step-process:

1. You need to reprogramme your unconscious mind to change certain behaviours
2. This instruction to change comes from your conscious mind
3. The unconscious mind learns the new way of doing things and produces new behaviour.

IMPORTANT
♥Before you do anything ensure you have read the first part of the book first, otherwise you are jumping too far ahead too soon, and this is not a good start. *So, if you haven't then go back and read it, and then get your pen and notebook.*

Significance of the Mind & Body working together

In earlier times, a few physicians dismissed digestive problems without any symptom of organic illness as being psychological. Scientists now think the mind and the body's operations are interconnected, as opposed to the past. Complex links are noted by doctors between the digestive and nervous systems; therefore, anything that influences one will concern the other due to the continuous exchange of electrical and chemical messages between the two. The original evidence relating the therapeutic power of the mind to our bodies is conveyed to us every day. Prayer or any kind of meditation genuinely soothes us, which in turn may assist us to face our routine stressors.

Nowadays, fitness specialists add on to this notion, essentially informing you which parts of your body and muscles are accountable, or 'connected' to which aspects of your daily living. This translates into physiology and psychology being attached together, and for those fitness enthusiasts planning workouts for clients this is a great issue to investigate in more detail. The fitness professionals are there to help the maintenance of the client's physical and 'mental' health, as fitness can aid physically, connecting 'psychologically'.

Willpower
Your attitude is shaped by your thoughts, feelings, and actions. It's really easy to

feel good when the going is good. The key to vibrant energy and a powerful attitude is to *make* yourself feel good, *especially* when the going is tough, and you don't feel good, or you don't want to feel good. Willpower is one of the tools you need to employ in order to resist the powerful cravings associated with food. The cravings will attempt to control you. It is your willpower, determination and self-discipline that you will use to fight back.

💡 Start by developing a strong willpower. Every person has the capacity to build up or strengthen his or her willpower by exercising it in times of need. Lifting weights develops muscles and exercising willpower makes it stronger. Add self-discipline in your life to become more aware of how you use your willpower in the course of all your daily activities.

💡 Making a positive mindset for weight loss
Keep in mind what you would like to hear about yourself from other people. Do you really need someone to fill you with positive thoughts and inspirations? Wouldn't you be able to do it yourself? Build your own positive thoughts and tell yourself everything that you would like to hear from others. Repeat those thoughts to yourself, everyday. You might find it strange initially, but after a while you might not even feel that you're doing it. In such a case, the maintenance of a healthy weight will be a near reality and not a distant dream.

Internal & external control

Gaining self-control
Would you rather be, <u>in</u> or <u>out</u> of control of your destiny?
Julian Rotters' most important concept (internal locus of control) states that internally controlled individuals assume that their own behaviours and actions are responsible for the consequences that happen to them. Alternatively externally controlled individuals believe that control is out of their hands. Barbara Engler (2009) highlights certain findings from research regarding internally controlled individuals such as they have more likelihood of achievement, more likely to know about the conditions that lead to good physical and emotional health, and more likely to assume more responsibility for their own behaviour.

I know which type of individual I'd rather be!

Barbara Engler (2009) also highlights the findings from research regarding externally controlled individuals too, such as they prefer not to make a choice, they are more anxious, depressed and vulnerable to stress. They also develop defensive strategies, always inviting failure. So it seems that the externally controlled type of people are the ones that would always find different ways of making excuses and giving reasons why they haven't achieved what they set out to do. Your job is to become more aware of your thinking habits, in order to develop a greater range of solutions for decision-making.

Other benefits of internal locus of control are:
- Better thinking skills
- Better memory to pick up new insights
- More likely to choose challenging tasks
- More willing to delay gratification and keep going when things get tough
- More likely to deal with and recover from illness
- Greater self-esteem and less anxiety
- Greater satisfaction with life and overall contentment.

Seems like this group of people are well on their way to success!

"Success is the ability to go from failure to failure without losing your enthusiasm."

- Winston Churchill

Your focus of control is what actually determines how the thinking procedure works about your fate. How these strategies work will be evident from the following:

Internal focus
If you want to be successful, you have to employ an internal focus of control. The first thing is to identify the internal focus of control, and if you have that, you would think that it is your action, thoughts and attitude that control your destiny. You think that the law of attraction has a huge effect on your goals. In other words, if you can see it, you think you can always make it. It is you who controls your own fate.

External focus
If you have an external focus of control, you will believe that your destiny is determined by external factors like luck, gods, sun signs, etc. However, this is not a very good success strategy.

If you focus on what it is you want to achieve by losing weight and think it out beforehand, then this change to the positive frame of mind will be easy. Create a 'wellness vision'. What are the benefits of losing weight that appeal to you? Think. Make this dream a vivid one, think it out carefully, all its aspects – physical, mental and aesthetic should be etched out in your mind. Then dwell on this vision and it will become your pattern of thought automatically. Dieting and exercising are important no doubt, but destroying the built up negativity inside you is no less important.

If you choose to switch over to a positive vision and remain committed to this vision, your subconscious will switch over from negative to positive. Repeat this and see whether you can lose weight this time – stay focused and dedicated to the cause.

The neuropsychology of weight control

<u>Winning the brain game</u>
Millions of people have a tough time controlling their weight as they strive to either maintain a diet regime, or keep thinking that they need to maintain one unless they have already given up trying. In today's world, a large section of people are suffering from obesity related problems, since they are not aware of the *three key* essentials for helping you to stick to high-level nutrition and continuously motivate yourself to do so.

These keys are:
1. Carbohydrate management
2. Timing your meals
3. Interactive self-hypnosis.

These can all help you to overcome the yo-yo weight gain syndrome and provide you with a healthy, energised body and a positive frame of mind. Interactive self-hypnosis can help you to win the brain game by helping you to control your subconscious mind, or at least know the way in which it works. Other than interactive self-hypnosis, active imagery, visualisation and NLP (neurolinguistic programming) can also help in weight control.

The subconscious mind, which is ruled by the right brain, perceives and stores active images that are visual, but actually includes all the senses. Specialised self-hypnosis education will help you understand how the mind really works; therefore, enable you to reach your goals easily. The interactive self-hypnosis technique is quite simple and can be learned and accessed by both children and adults.
However, these techniques vary according to clients, since different individuals react in different ways to their surroundings and are motivated to respond to specific images and metaphors. The duration of these hypnotic sessions can also vary according to the needs of the individual concerned.

These sessions are generally divided into the following:
• Induction – that includes deepening techniques
• The metaphoric elements being delivered
• The process of emerging.

Self-motivation and persistence is stressed upon and given special importance to, and this in turn arms you with better weight loss management skills, and such techniques fall under the broad category of neuropsychology. Interactive self-hypnosis increases your focusing abilities; therefore, enables you to stick to the necessary regimen and improve your body image and self-esteem. If you are obese there is a tendency to get frightened while trying to come to terms with your new self that emerges having gone through the weight loss program. Fear and anxiety might arise from you, not having imagined yourself before in such a way, and interactive self-hypnosis sessions help in these cases to release this fear and anxiety.

Neuropsychology helps you to develop a multifaceted approach towards weight; therefore, making the process more enjoyable for you. It helps you control your mind and body better, and helps you taste success in a far more relaxed and easier manner. You can possess a healthy body with a great digestive and metabolic system and an increased level of immunity. Not only will your stress levels be decreased, but also neuropsychology of weight control will help you to win the brain game, enabling you to lead a healthier and fuller life.

Your approach to the psychology of weight loss
The whole world is currently faced with a critical situation of succumbing to the epidemic of obesity and blood sugar. Your boat will sink if you weigh it down with your psychological barriers related to weight loss by loading it with statistics of grams, calories and pounds. You want to feel better and stronger by losing some weight, but you do not know the right path to being successful in your endeavour. In order to prevent your general health from going down the drain, you must adopt these two steps:

Step 1 – Get rid of your hang-ups!
It is not really difficult for you to start exercising. You should concentrate more upon the positive aspect of exercise instead of unconsciously resisting the idea. Exercise resistance refers to the conscious or unconscious blocking out of participation in a programme that demands regular activities. This might result from bitter past experiences, which turns you into being apathetic towards exercise and healthy food. More often than not these thoughts prevent you from religiously following an exercise programme. The root of resenting exercise travels far deeper than just disliking the effort it takes to carry it out, and this resentment will only make a rebel out of you.

What you really need to do is accept exercise as a part of your life, as something that is as important as brushing your teeth or combing your hair. Resentment comes hand in hand with denial, vanity and laziness. Success can never be measured by virtue of its numerical or statistical value, but by the ways in which you keep growing in due course of the process. First and foremost you must never be afraid of failure, and you must keep in mind that perfection can never really be achieved permanently, as it is but an illusion.

Step 2 – Changing your beliefs about life, food and exercise
You need to unearth the roots of the things you are concerned with, and you need to come to terms with your attitude towards exercise and eating.

- Do you live under the illusion that you are very much acquainted with your thought procedures?
- Does reality elude you?

You should also keep in mind to never compare yourself with the performances of others either. Goals, no matter how many you achieve or score, will always be there, and what really counts is improving yourself since you are the best judge of your own standards. The psychology of weight loss has both negative as well as positive sides; however, when it comes to the negative aspect, you might overburden yourself with high expectations that leads to setting yourself up for failure. Ultimately this can prove to be extremely harmful.

Suggestion

If you really want to change your food and exercise habits, you need to get to the heart of the matter and discover the reasons behind your behaviour. In this context your beliefs and faith have a huge and important role to play. Your beliefs and faith stem from your core values that influence an essential part of your life.

You can overcome a great deal of your limitations if you can adjust your beliefs accordingly, which lie deep within you. Only your beliefs can stand against your successful carrying out of exercise programmes, and your beliefs need to be changed if necessary. You can never have everything easy, and to get to where you need to be takes a great deal of time, energy and effort on your part.

Your core, emotional values will ultimately determine your choices. Once you identify your heartfelt desires, you can use them to create a healthy lifestyle that reflects your best self. Your deepest values can be summoned to keep you on track, especially when you are facing temptations and distractions. They can also serve as your compass when you go astray.

Be aware of letting weight loss take over your life. Losing weight is a fantastic achievement, but it is just another challenge in life...as is battling with your thoughts, emotions and behaviours. Recapture those moments of how you were when you had it good.

Values

Act on your (morals and) values
We are emotional beings with the ability to rationalise; we are not rational beings with emotions. In a nutshell 'values' are words that depict what is most important to you in your life.

We have given you examples of some of these values. There are too many to list them all, but you should take the opportunity to write yours down too and put them in order of importance to you.
 1. Self-respect
 2. Worthiness
 3. Usefulness
 4. Sacrifice
 5. Pride
 6. Trustworthiness
 7. Recognition
 8. Inspiration
 9. Happiness

38

10. Decisiveness
11. Cheerfulness
12. Acceptance.

♥Task 16
Act on your morals and values by first of all writing them down below. Yours are:

1. ....
2. ....
3. ....
4. ....
5. ....
6. ....
7. ....
8. ....
9. ....
10. ....

Always remember your core values and what you bring to the table as the unique person that you are. Avoid letting the whole weight loss journey damage your sense of yourself. Be clear about your values regarding your overall health. Choosing to act on your values will strengthen your sense of yourself as a capable person.

As you progress from day-to-day, you will not only value your life more, but also every moment. If you are willing to remain diligently committed to your emotional values, you can be confident that you will succeed in realising your health and fitness goals.

And when you do, maybe some of you will go one step further and give support to family and friends so that they can join you in becoming healthier and happier.

Respect & self-worth

Respect. Life. The air that we breathe. The human body and each moment. How would you rate your *self-worth*?

You Only Live Once
Life is not a rehearsal, we know this...and although that can also mean 'live for today' it does mean that if you want to live a longer life without pain and suffering you must respect yourself more, especially your body. Too many people use this prospect to poison themselves into thinking it's OK to eat and drink what they want and to excess.

Doing this quite frankly is setting yourself up for an early exit.
You don't have to be religious to understand that a higher being (God, Allah, Buddha, the universe, etc.) is watching over us to ensure that we are each loved dearly

and we can achieve anything we manifest i.e. put our minds too. Whether you believe this or not is irrelevant, but what is certain is that love must start by loving yourself first. Self-love provides you with self-esteem, which in turn provides you with self-confidence, a level of motivation and all the other attributes needed for success.

Acceptance that you are who you are is also a contributory factor to the above. Yes you are overweight, but you don't have to be. Who says so? Just respect the fact that each of us are different physically yet very much the same internally and physiologically. Your self-image can change for the better or worse and this is very much up to you in the sense that however you think of yourself, this image will then be portrayed to the world.

For example, you have a bad day but, until you change this thought process these feelings have a tendency to attract similar people or things into your life. You must have had a good day too right? Nonetheless, have you learnt to know and feel the difference between the two? And have you witnessed the type of things or people that you attract? Respecting yourself starts from within, what you say and do is all a by-product of what you have originally thought or felt. Your attitude creates your actions, but are they positive and will they benefit you on your journey? Respecting yourself first and foremost allows you to respect others, and this in turn will get you respect from those around you.

A dietician, holistic therapist or psychologist's specialised suggestions will aid you to tide over your feelings of loathing and repulsion. After intimately discussing with them, chalk out an improvement plan and define your personal values, which are appropriate for you and relevant to your specific goals. Only after learning about your internal self can you surely uncover the true strength of your self-esteem and energy to completely achieve your goals, irrespective of what people think or say.

Self-efficacy
Self-efficacy is your belief that you can change what you want to change, no matter what the circumstances are. For example that you feel confident you can eat a healthy diet even when you feel your time is limited, at a table when others are eating a dessert, or quite simply when you are bored or unhappy and you want to snap out of it and start to feel better.

Your self-esteem

Most people are unhappy with their bodies; therefore, unable to accept the way they are. What doesn't help is the portrayal of the so-called body ideals of various celebrities and supermodels, and this is one of the many reasons why people are unable to overcome eating disorders.

Feeling deprived

As you are well aware, you desire the foods that you love more when you are denied them. Therefore, if you give in to temptation due to such restrictions, you break your plan that puts you right back to square one. Unfortunately, such prohibited food types are extremely accessible and advertised as such. However, after giving in to temptation a devastating guilt is felt and consequently a low self-esteem.

Be aware of how grateful you are for 'life'

You are stronger than you think and having an awareness of any negativity, self-doubt and denial you may have had in the past, will help you to move forward in a successful and positive manner. Being 'in the now' is something that takes time to master, especially if you daydream a lot or have many things going on in your life.

However, being more aware and paying attention to you maintaining a healthy life is something that is definitely extremely important to take with you on your new journey.

♥ Task 17

Ask for encouragement from:
- Your friends
- Your family
- Seek encouragement from a role model.

You must ensure that your role model is realistic i.e. not someone who has been paid to be in a magazine, who has been airbrushed, or only lost weight temporarily. Your role model must be someone who has genuinely lost weight for themselves, maybe after a pregnancy or a health scare, etc. But it must have been permanent weight loss success. Your encouragement comes from being able to tell yourself, "If he or she can do it, so can I" and then you can believe it.

Remember the point that we are trying to make here is that a large part of the weight loss battle is psychological. Weight loss is difficult, no one is denying that. But it is more than possible and healthy mindful changes will positively ensure you reach your goals. Believing you can lose weight is essential to your long-term success.

Turn your positive thoughts into reality and success; only you can change it, nobody else. Adjust your mind into thinking about what you need to do…and get going. When your mind is truly focused on the journey and focused on success you will achieve all that you've ever dreamt about.

Do you actually know what you are capable of achieving?

If you make a plan to succeed and actually believe that at the end of it you will lose weight, then what's the problem? So many times we fall short of our desires due to self-doubt and fear of failure, but you are capable of achieving exactly what you want. Perhaps somewhere along the way you have lost your way? Now its time to get back on track!

"Stop saying *'I wish'* and start saying *'I will."*

- +PositiveMed

♥Task 18
Write down all your accomplishments to date, everything you have done in your life. For example, it could be given birth successfully, captain of the school team, saved up to buy my own car, etc.

Overcoming barriers

Get the job done, no matter what
So what can you do to ensure that you do what you set out to do? Having a selection of punishments is a good idea, but these will have to be pre-set in order for them to work.
1. Tell everyone what you are doing in order to make you 100% accountable
2. With the help of your support (a family member, friend or our website) set yourself certain punishment(s) just in case, but it has to be someone who will without fail initiate the punishment.

Your list of punishments could be something financial, something that goes against your beliefs or something that is embarrassing for you or anything similar.

For example, your punishment could be to:
*   register you for a fitness event i.e. a competition or a running event
*   donate your money to a cause that you do not support
*   anything similar.

Temptation
Most of us get punished after an event has occurred, but according to Richard Gross (1992) punishment that is consistently given before a misdeed results in high resistance to temptation. So if like most people you were to classify exercise as a punishment this would explain why their temptation to eating and drinking unhealthy foods is significant. Gross also points out something equally important; is the finding that, when *reasons* are given, the timing of punishment becomes irrelevant. This explains why when you look at the sweet trolley you just think about the effort you have just put in at the gym.

Be resilient
Being prepared for knock backs is one thing, and therefore your expectations should not be too high, but if you focus your mind on progressing (no matter what) all will be well. Your ability to weather any storm that comes your way is an essential part to any programme and requires a great deal of perseverance and flexibility. The

42

strategy you decide to use may not always work, so you may need to continually review, adapt and monitor your plan accordingly. You will always need to maintain positive yet constructive thoughts in order to keep the vision of your successful future at the forefront of your mind.

Task checklist

Part 2: Psychology

☐ ♥ Task 10

Address your lifestyle patterns.

☐ ♥ Task 11

Work out what it is that's bothering you…

☐ ♥ Task 12

Lifestyle Challenge 1 - Positive self-talk phrases.

☐ ♥ Task 13

It is also important to understand the type of pattern that you associate with food.

☐ ♥ Task 14

Stress is one of the most common killers of human beings. So from this moment on, promise yourself that you will take each moment, each second, every minute, hour and day in your stride, and live each breath as if it were your last.

☐ ♥ Task 15

Attempt the following tasks to help you with the questions about perception.

☐ ♥ Task 16

Act on your morals and values by first of all writing them down below.

☐ ♥ Task 17

Ask for encouragement.

☐ ♥ Task 18

Write down all your accomplishments to date, everything you have done in your life example. it could be given birth successfully, captain of the school team, saved up to buy my own car, etc.

"There is no passion to be found playing small - in settling for a life that is less than the one you are capable of living."

- Nelson Mandela

Part 3: NUTRITION

Does your body need a spring clean?

Somebody once told me that weight loss is 80% nutrition and 20% exercise, so if that's the case where does 'psychology' come into play?

As mentioned previously, for you to be psychologically better off you need to have all the answers in front of you. For permanent weight loss success you need to think of the 'mind' and the 'body' collectively; therefore, you need to know about how you can change not just your thought patterns, but also your food and exercise choices too.

So if you know what foods are best for you and what exercise you must do then you will almost certainly be psychologically better off on your path to permanent weight loss success.

Before you start to consume healthy nutritious foods however, it's always a good idea to have a good cleanse to get rid of any impurities first.

Cleansing has many benefits such as:
- It normalises your digestion and your metabolism by eliminating acid wastes and negative microforms
- It detoxifies your blood and tissues and generally regains your alkaline balance.

A world-renowned microbiologist and nutritionist named Dr Robert Young (2002) explains that "a cleanse is basically a liquid feast where you get 20 times more food than you would generally." A cleanse is recommended to all those who have subjected their body to a typical western (acidic) diet. He goes on to say that "a cleanse can last anything from 24 hours to 10 days depending on the person and their situation."

As always consultation with your healthcare professional is advised.

So what do you already know about 'How to lose weight'?

- Do you know that alcohol is laden with calories?
- What do you feel about late night snacking?
- Do you know which carbs are good and who needs them most?
- Should you know more about glucose and insulin?

♥Task 19
Write down what you definitely know to be true. For example:

44

- My mother always taught me that vegetables are good for me; therefore, if I fill up on these then I can have a reduced amount of meat or carbohydrate i.e. not too much potatoes or rice
- I also know that salads are good for me but I know that I need to be aware of salad dressings unless they are prepared with healthy fats
- I know that food portion sizes are important.

"For good health and longevity, educating children in their home environment is the priority of all parents. It is even more important to teach children about good food choices outside of the home."

- Wellness FitCoach

Don't always believe what you are told
Buying low fat, sugar free, diet this, diet that…isn't always the way to go. So start reading the back of packets and comparing if it is actually what it is advertised as.

"Integrity is the key to a successful life, so whatever you decide to do each day have the courage to say no from time to time, especially if it's the right thing to do."

- Wellness FitCoach

Your current nutrition

Questions to ask yourself about your current nutrition:
- How healthy is a 'low fat' diet?
- Are you eating enough?
- Do you skip meals?
- Are you lacking in fibre?

According to Patrick Holford (2006) weight gain is a common reaction to foods we're intolerant to, and eliminating such foods can lead to dramatic weight loss. Below are some of the problems that can be encountered, with the top three even making you feel and look fatter:
- Water retention (can also be due to a lack of essential fats, too much sugar and salt in the body)
- Bloating
- Puffiness
- Aches and pains
- Headaches
- Fatigue
- Mood swings
- Skin and digestive conditions.

45

He goes on to advise that 'dramatic changes are likely to be seen once these foods have been singled out and eliminated.'

The 10 most common allergy-provoking foods according to Holford are:
1. Cow's milk
2. Yeast
3. Wheat
4. Gliadin grains (in gluten)
5. Oats
6. Eggs
7. Beans
8. Nuts
9. Shellfish
10. White fish.

What could current food choices be doing to your insides?
If you are not a vegetarian or vegan then chances are that 26% of your calories are from animal products alone. So what does this mean?
- Cancer promoting
- Inflammation
- Cellular growth
- Excess calories
- Insulin-like growth factor? (Insulin receptors get clogged up from olive oils and fats, which eventually leads to diabetes).

Facts you may not know about poor food choices
- Too much food is being advertised and consumed that is un-nutritional
- Most seafood is polluted
- Convenience foods (sugar and fatty choices) are deemed as affordable, but they are sky-high in calories.

Building a shield for your brain
You could be losing your mind for the sake of a burger; if you are, you can help yourself by reducing your intake of the following:
- Most animal products
- Saturated fats (in cheese, milk, yogurt and even chicken too)
- Trans fats
- Partially hydrogenated oils.

If your (bad) cholesterol remains high, you risk doubling your normal age i.e. if you are 40 years of age your body will feel 80 years.

How excess fat can affect your body

An overweight person having increased levels of inflammation is a known scientific fact; to this day the tracing of a part of this inflammation to the fat itself is carried out by various studies. Fat cells churn out low-grade systemic inflammation proteins called cytokines in overweight people.

Pro-inflammatory omega-6s are found a lot in refined vegetable oils like corn and safflower. Adding that low-level inflammation may contribute to disease, location is important for excess body fat. The fat surrounding the abdomen is the greatest source of inflammation.

Astrup A. and colleagues completed a study at the Research Department of Human Nutrition & LMC in Denmark, of the role of dietary fat in the body.

The study concluded that:
- Fewer calories in a low-fat diet with high proteins and fibre-rich carbohydrates, primarily from different vegetables, fruits and whole grains, is more highly satisfying than fatty foods.
- The most beneficial effect on blood lipids and levels of blood pressure are seen in this diet composition providing good sources of vitamins, minerals, trace elements and fibre.

In subjects of normal weight, reducing dietary fat without restricting total energy intake prevents weight gain. This same diet produces a weight loss in overweight subjects (which is highly significant for public health).
(A. Astrup, G.K. Grunwald, E.L. Melanson, W.H.M. Saris & J.O. Hill, 2000)

Biochemical consequences
Since caveman times, the digestive system has evolved from consuming lean protein, fruits and vegetables to us now consuming large amounts of refined grains, bread and pasta. Although these food types were not around 8000 years ago, from a genetic standpoint we are struggling to adapt to a diet high in grains, and we are setting ourselves up to suffering adverse biochemical consequences.

Carbohydrate rich foods and glucose
Our bodies are open to various diseases and poor health due to Eicosanoids; these are types of (pancreatic) hormones and by-products of normal metabolic processes. Insulin is not actually the culprit in producing 'bad' eicosanoids, because it is necessary for life itself and directly supplies energy by transferring glucose from the blood into the cells of the body (including muscle cells) for availability as an energy substrate.

Adverse effects on your health and physiology
Throughout a day's pattern of food intake and physical activity, insulin levels must fluctuate within a 24 hour period in order to maintain normal blood glucose levels.

47

Avoid poor performance from low carb diets

Low carbohydrate diets could easily lead to muscle glycogen depletion and protein loss, which would not be good for you at all. However, calorie deficient diets will always result in weight loss, but a diet that's combined with exercise will require an adequate intake of carbs in order to replenish glycogen stores to maintain your energy levels. This in turn results in a higher percentage of weight loss for you and assists you over the long-term for permanent results.

Low 'total' calorie diets

If you want to lose weight and maintain that same weight afterwards, the answer comes from medium-high carbohydrate diets. However, you must bear in mind that if your diet has a high glycaemic index it can be converted readily to fat if your overall energy intake is high. Confused? Read on...

Combining carbs and fat in your diet to burn fat

A wide range of dietary patterns may be acceptable when you are trying to lose weight, but the following is important to know for best results:

- Too much fat in the diet results in a negative carbohydrate balance over the period of an exercise session; therefore, not allowing for further exercise
- Carbs are required by your muscles in order for your body to sustain any type of physical activity
- If a high-carbohydrate diet is consumed, your body finds it difficult to burn fat even at lower intensities.

Solution

When you consume a high level of 'good fats', a moderate amount of carbohydrates and workout at a moderate intensity, fat becomes the main source of energy.

Facts about healthier type foods

A variety of healthy foods are high in micronutrients per calorie; therefore, there is no risk of overeating in calories.

Wellness FitCoach rule

Avoid the 3 white poisons:
1. *Sugar* – Sweet foods like cakes, biscuits, cookies, sweets, etc.
2. *Flour* – Anything in a pastry base i.e. pies, pasties, croissants, etc.
3. *Salt* – Processed foods in a tin, additional salt on your meals, etc. as this leads to high blood pressure (BP) and can increase your stress levels too.

Sugar – one item to avoid!

Did you know that sugar is a leading cause of illness? Here are some examples:
- Cancer – sugar actually feeds cancer cells
- Diabetes
- Obesity

- Heart disease
- Arthritis
- Gallstones
- Dental problems.

Sugar-fix calories

Many 'high-carbohydrate' foods, notably biscuits, cakes, pies and candy bars are laden with fat; therefore, stepping up the intake of these consumables are a sure way of padding out your body with bloated adipose cells.
(Medicine and science in sports and exercise, 1994).

Sugar is not necessary in our diet. In fact sugar is *toxic and addictive.* Many people actually eat sugar as a food i.e. by consuming copious amounts of liquid food by way of soda, and added to a burger meal this can add up to a whopping ½ lb. of sugar per day.

Here's how:
- Drink
- Burger
- Bun
- Sauce
- Fries.

It all adds up and this is what ultimately leads to obesity and an increased risk of diabetes.

Don't be conned by diet foods and drinks

According to Gill Paul (2009) low fat, low calorie diet foods are designed by manufacturers to satisfy taste buds. She goes on to mention that rather than fat, and in order to taste similar they often rely on the following additives and chemicals:
- Monosodium glutamate (MSG)
- Emulsifiers
- Flavour enhances
- Artificial sweeteners
- Sugar.

Many of these types of foods and drink also contain trans-fats which can cause heart disease, obesity and many other health problems.

Fructose

Fructose is another name for sugar, which is hidden in virtually every processed food. It tricks your body into gaining weight by fooling your metabolism, as it turns off your body's appetite-control system. Fructose does not appropriately stimulate insulin, which in turn does not suppress ghrelin (the 'hunger hormone') and doesn't stimulate leptin (the 'satiety hormone'), which together result in your eating more and developing insulin resistance. It's very easy to sabotage yourself with sugary foods and beverages, especially those that contain fructose. This includes so-called 'healthy' beverages like 'vitamin water', energy drinks and similar types of sports and recovery drinks.

Fructose also rapidly leads to weight gain and abdominal obesity (beer belly), decreased HDL, increased LDL, elevated triglycerides, elevated blood sugar, and high blood pressure i.e. classic metabolic syndrome.

How serious do you want it to sound?
All of these refined foods not only age us, they also make us toxic, and can and will lead to an early death.

Why not white bread or flour?
In general, wholemeal bread contains twice as much iron, three times as much zinc, and four times as much fibre as basic white bread.

What does milling wheat into white flour do?
- It removes the outer bran coat and wheatgerm
- This process loses most of the thiamin, niacin and iron
- Millers are legally obliged to replace B vitamins lost, but do they do that?

What does wholemeal mean to you?
Wholemeal contains the wholewheat kernel and fibre-rich bran, and it provides the following:
- B group vitamins (thiamine and niacin)
- Vitamin E, iron, selenium and other minerals, phytonutrients and bran
- It's an important source of roughage (insoluble fibre).

Start as you mean to go on. So, do you now have some new items on your shopping list, healthy items that you can realistically consume without question?

A brief overview about eating

When you eat food, your blood glucose levels rise. Your body reacts by producing insulin to steer the glucose into working muscles and into the liver. Sometimes there is a problem with this if you consume more glucose than your body needs and diabetes is the outcome. What can you do? Eat foods that release glucose slower into the blood such as *Low GI*.

♥Task 20
Without healthy nutrition, your weight loss is doomed for failure, and because our philosophy does not include negativity we task you with doing the following:
- Go in your kitchen and take out all your crisps, biscuits, cakes, sweets, soda drinks, anything wrapped in pastry and/or covered in sugar, and anything else you feel is not healthy. Give it all to someone who doesn't

have money or someone you feel does not need to worry about weight gain. Tell them they are helping you if they accept it from you.
- Reduce or stop consuming the following: (all the above) plus everything you deem to include in their ingredients 'the 3 white poisons' – 1. White refined sugar, 2. White refined flour, 3. Salt.

IMPORTANT
More time and determination is required from you with many fad diets that are out there today and you have to follow them through which requires more effort from you.

Most diets, etc. can be:
- Impractical
- Expensive
- Unsociable
- Limiting with choice.

Extra effort and time is needed to plan and prepare personal meals and snacks based on an exact prescribed formula. Cutting your calories strictly limits your food choices. Therefore, your choice of 'healthy' snacks needs to be unlimited.

Self-sabotage vs self-control

Although having a low body weight can be helpful for your health, caution is urged if success comes from using extreme strategies. Restricting food intake is the reason 80% of traditional weight loss approaches fail, and in some cases it would be difficult in normal everyday life to actually achieve some of the formulas set out in certain 'low calorie' programmes. Also, a life of obsessive eating behaviours only leads to yo-yo dieting, chronic hunger and mood swings, and these are all due to extreme weight loss techniques, which is what we want to avoid.

Most participants of the diet plans that are on the market today put themselves in a state of energy deprivation due to there being too much restriction of calories. Also, these diets seldom calculate for energy expenditure through exercise that is a major component to long-term weight loss success. Drastic measures to lose weight can also lead to dehydration and reduced energy levels, which in turn, leads to poor exercise performance.
So it's no wonder you never feel up to it when it comes to getting motivated for exercise. In the long run this all leads to reducing your mojo (self-esteem, confidence, motivation, etc.), which is what we want to avoid. Engaging in some form of exercise and eating a healthy diet is an effective way of controlling weight and raising self-esteem, but it is important to avoid developing obsessive thoughts about the word 'diet'.

51

Evidence suggests that the majority of those who diet to lose weight fail to keep the weight off over an extended period and have a higher weight gain in the future compared with individuals who do not diet. (I Journal of Obesity, 1994). In an ideal world you would eat healthily without any difficulty and maintain a healthy weight, but first of all and in order for this to happen we must ensure that you learn strategies to maintain a healthy weight without dieting at all.

Nutrient-dense foods = longevity

In order to reach and maintain a healthy weight, you must make yourself aware of energy-dense foods, and therefore most of the foods you consume should be low energy density ones.

<u>What is energy density?</u>
It is defined as the number of calories per serving of food. For example, high fat foods often have high energy density i.e. lots of calories in a small amount of food, and this is the main reason why you never feel full or satisfied when you eat fast food and the reason why you are hungry shortly afterwards. In order to acquire all the vitamins, minerals and phytonutrients that your body requires, you need a variety of different food types. Your portion sizes should also fulfill the minimum nutritional recommendations.

It would be very wise to teach yourself how to *graze on your food instead of gorging on it* as this is very important regarding the amount of carbohydrate you eat which has the biggest influence on your blood glucose levels after meals and likewise your weight loss attempts. The average diet creates a 'toxic hunger' that in turn leads to an increased desire for calories due to never being satisfied, which is why these foods seem addictive because you are constantly trying to get full. More importantly though, this method of eating is like a drug and makes it pretty impossible for you to lose weight.

On a good note, when you implement our nutritional strategies into your life you will quite frankly turn your diet up on it's head and you will put an end to dieting once and for all. If you think that only 10% of the average persons calories come from vegetables, fruits, beans, seeds and nuts. So if we can flip that on its head so that you are consuming a hell of a lot more, then you can only imagine the long-term health benefits.

<u>So what do you have to eat?</u>
Nutrient-dense foods that are rich in the following:
- ✓ Vitamins
- ✓ Minerals
- ✓ Phytochemicals
- ✓ Antioxidants
- ✓ Low in calories.

What happens internally when you start to consume nutrient-dense foods?
- You flood your cells and tissues with protective substances
- You naturally guide your body back to its ideal weight
- You no longer have hunger pangs or have feelings of deprivation.

What are the long-term benefits of consuming nutrient-dense foods?
- Dramatic weight loss
- Optimal overall health
- Longevity.

So, to conquer weight loss forever, you need to stop eating sugar, refined carbo-hydrates and animal products i.e. foods that are low in micronutrients, contain no beneficial phytochemicals and have addictive properties.

Supplements

Even the healthiest diet may not contain the key nutrients that your body needs to function at optimal level. Fat burning supplements stabilise your appetite, sugar cravings and help fine-tune your metabolism. In the first 3 months of changing your eating habits Patrick Holford (2006) recommends the following supplements, espe-cially if you are prone to sugar cravings and have poor appetite control.

In addition to a high strength multi-vitamin and multi-mineral and 1000mg of vita-min C a day a combination of the following is recommended:
1. Hydroxycitric acid (HCA) – 30 mins before lunch and dinner
2. 5-hydroxytryptophan (HTP) – twice daily with fruit
3. Chromium – twice daily with mid-morning and afternoon snacks.

A good multivitamin and mineral tablet will supply antioxidants, below is a list of other nutrients that are critical to the detoxification process:
- Magnesium
- Potassium
- Frolic acid
- Zinc
- Selenium
- Molybdenum
- Beta carotene
- Biotin
- B-complex vitamins
- Choline.

Basic guidelines
With any food pyramid you must have a sturdy base, a high point, and a triangular shape that gradually narrows to its highest point as it cleverly reduces the foods that you should consume in moderation.

Drinks

8 to 10 glasses of filtered or sparkling water (per day, before and after each meal and snack), Green or black tea in moderation. Fat-free instant chocolate, decaffeinated coffee, sugar-free soft drinks, skimmed milk (GI 32), sugar-free fruit juice, decaffeinated tea and freshly squeezed juices.

Fruits and vegetables

Fruits and vegetables should be amongst the foods you eat the most of, and therefore these should form the sturdy base of your pyramid. You should try and consume at least three fruits a day (60 calories each) and more if you can, 4 or more servings of non-starchy vegetables (25 calories each) may be consumed in unlimited amounts, and for weight loss purposes these are very filling and will likewise leave your appetite 100% satisfied. Most non-starchy vegetables aren't tested (on the GI scale) because a person would have to eat so much to get 50 grams of carbohydrate for the test, but on the other hand, some non-starchy vegetables have more sugar than others.

Carbohydrates

These should also be at the base of your pyramid, and should consist of whole grain pasta, bread, rice, and cereals. You should try and eat 4-8 servings of whole grains.

Protein and dairy

These should be at the next level of your pyramid. You should try and eat 3-7 servings of seafood, lean meat and poultry, eggs, beans and peas, soy products, and unsalted nuts and seeds. Eat fish and plant sources of protein more often and in greater variety in place of some meat and poultry.

Eggs

Ensure you buy omega-3 eggs, which are eggs laid by chickens that have been fed with omega-3 rich food, as these are lower in saturated fat.

Meats

Should be lean cuts, or you should trim off any visible fat, back bacon, beef (lean cuts), chicken breast (skinless), minced beef (extra lean), lean ham and turkey.

Fish

A typical portion should fit into the palm of your hand and be about as thick. All fresh, frozen or canned fish and seafood is allowed, to include: Bass, calamari, clams, cod, crab, crayfish, dory, haddock, halibut, herring, lobster, mackerel, oysters, salmon, sardines, scallops, snapper, sole, swordfish, trout, tuna and tuna tinned in water where available.

For digestion purposes you should focus on eating protein with carbohydrates.

Fats & Oils
These should be towards the top of your pyramid and likewise eaten in limited amounts. You should try and eat 3-5 servings of fats (olive oil, canola oil, avocados, almonds, flax seed, hazelnuts, macadamia nuts, mayonnaise (fat-free), margarine (polyunsaturated), rapeseed oil and salad dressings that are fat-free.

http://EzineArticles.com/119399
http://www.dailymail.co.uk/health/article-152012/The-GI-diet-List-low-glycaemic-foods.html#ixzz2a3lTg3jg

Are GI foods and exercise the key to long-term weight loss success?
There are many fad diets around, and many various ways and means of losing weight, however a formula that seems to work the best is the combination between the GI (Glycemic Index) diet combined with exercise. In short you should aim to include more foods with a low glycemic index into your diet, your body will digest these foods slowly leaving you feeling full for longer and allow you to eat less calories without feeling hungry. As an added bonus, when you add a low GI food to a meal it will lower the glycemic index of the whole meal. Overall, combined with exercise you will be able to lose weight and sustain your weight loss more permanently.

What do low glycemic foods actually do?
- They release their glucose into your body at a slower rate
- They allow you to maintain more stable energy levels for longer
- They ensure you stop producing more glucose than your body can actually use.

These foods prevent you from:
- Gaining fat, because they reprogram your body to burn fat more rapidly
- Suffering from food cravings.

Your aim should be to get to know what is high or low GI when you are out shopping in the supermarket, and also when you eat out at restaurants. After 21 days this simply becomes a habit and the new way that you shop/eat/and live. Changing this important part of your life then becomes permanent. Besides assisting you to lose weight, when you combine low GI foods with exercise this also provides you with many added health benefits too.

Putting it all on your plate – Low GI

(Summarised best by R.A. Price, 2008).

The number listed next to each food is its Glycemic Index (GI). This is a value obtained by monitoring a person's blood sugar after eating the food. For simplicity we have only listed the Low GI foods for you – low GI being 55 or less.

55

Breakfast Cereals

All bran (UK/Aus)	30
Natural Muesli	40
All bran (US)	50
Oat bran	50
Rolled Oats	51
Special K (UK/Aus)	54

Staples (foods that are stored easily & eaten often

Pearled Barley	22
Wheat tortilla	30
Spaghetti	32
Egg Fettuccini	32
Yam	35
Meat R	39
Instant Noodles	47
Sweet Potatoes	48
Brown Rice	50
White long grain rice	50
Tortellini (Cheese)	50
Buckwheat	51
Wheat Pasta Shapes	54
New Potatoes	54

Bread

Soya and Linseed	36
Heavy Mixed Grain	45
Wholegrain Pumpernickel	46
Sourdough Rye	48
Whole Wheat	49
Sourdough Wheat	54

Snacks & Sweet Foods

Hummus	6
Peanuts	14
Walnuts	15
Nuts and Raisins	21
Cashew Nuts	24
Nutella	33
Snickers Bar (high fat)	41
Milk Chocolate	42
Corn Chips	42
Sponge Cake	46
Nut & Seed Muesli Bar	49
Jam	51
Oatmeal Crackers	55

Legumes/Beans - (Canned beans tend to have a higher Glycemic Index)

Soy beans	18
Lentils, Red	21
Lentils, Green	30
Haricot/Navy Beans	31
Yellow Split Peas	32
Butter Beans	36
Chick Peas	42
Pinto Beans	45
Black-eyed Beans	50
Kidney Beans (canned)	52

Vegetables

Broccoli	10
Cabbage	10
Mushrooms	10
Chillies	10
Lettuce	10
Red Peppers	10
Onions	10
Green Beans	15
Tomatoes	15
Cauliflower	15
Eggplant/Aubergine	15
Raw Carrots	16
Frozen Green Peas	39
Boiled Carrots	41
Frozen Sweet Corn	47

Fruits

Cherries	22
Plums	24
Grapefruit	25
Peaches	28
Prunes	29
Peaches, canned in natural juice	30
Banana, under ripe	30
Dried Apricots	31
Apples	34
Oranges	40
Strawberries	40
Pears	41
Coconut Milk	41
Coconut	45
Grapes	46
Kiwi Fruit	47

Mangoes	51 (average)
Banana, overripe	52
Apricot fruit spread	55 (reduced sugar)

Fruit juices
Tomato Juice	38
Orange Juice	41
Carrot Juice	43
Pineapple Juice	46
Grapefruit Juice	48

Dairy
Artificially Sweetened Yoghurt	23
Whole milk	31
Skimmed milk	32
Sweetened yoghurt	33
Custard	35
Chocolate milk	42
Soy Milk	44

Information provided by the University of Sydney/
http://lowcarbdiets.about.com/od/whattoeat/a/glycemicindlist.htm
R. Gallup, The G.I. (Glycemic Index) Diet

💡Tips during mealtimes
Choose lots of low GI carbohydrates as your staples during the week. Eat plenty of fruits and vegetables from this group, but think of pasta and rice as side orders (1/4 plate), rather than the main food on your plate.

Go easy on lower GI foods like chocolate and nuts, which are high in fat and calories, especially if you are trying to lose weight, so save them for the occasional treat.

IMPORTANT
It is important for you not to focus exclusively on GI but to think about the overall balance of your meals, which should be low in fat, salt and sugar and contain plenty of fruit and vegetables.

Your nutritious overhaul

Food choices and food training
💡From now on concentrate fully on the food that you eat i.e. think only of the taste, the smell, and the very enjoyment of eating, emotions and other things related to the meal. This will assist you in two ways:

1. It will focus your attention to the present act; therefore, allow you to be satisfied with whatever you are eating
2. It might also keep your weight in check, as in most weight loss schemes one significant factor is that you need to be conscious of your entire meal process.

♥ Task 21
Write down some of your current food choices that you feel could be better. Example:
1. I eat fast food regularly, so I could reduce this by cooking my own meals
2. I drink a lot of soda, so I could reduce this and start to drink more water.

Foods for weight loss

Below is a list of different types of foods that have been researched by David Grotto (2007) whose findings discovered that they all assisted with weight loss in one way or another. The evidence suggests that the following food types help weight loss in the following ways:
- Almonds (help improve satiety)
- Apples (three per day helped individuals lose more weight than those who didn't eat them. Also, diabetics had smaller spikes in glucose after eating)
- Pulses and legumes (bean-eaters are less obese than people who don't include beans in their daily diet)
- Buckwheat (good for appetite control, people feel fuller after consumption compared to other grains)
- Carob (has fat burning properties)
- Eggs (have 'hunger fighting power' and if eaten in the morning can lead to reduced calorie consumption for the rest of the day)
- Figs (makes you feel full faster and slows absorption of calories, also may reduce the risk of developing type II diabetes)
- Grapefruit (one half before meals helped people lose a significant amount of weight improved insulin resistance)
- Grapes (grape seed extract may limit absorption and accumulation of dietary fat cells)
- Low fat dairy (studies have linked it with better weight management)
- Millet (can decrease levels of insulin sensitivity and manage glucose better)
- Oats (whole grain intake can help maintain a healthy weight, provides a feeling of fullness, lowers risk for developing type II diabetes)
- Oranges (white layer of orange curbs appetite and suppresses hunger levels for up to four hours after eating. Studies also show that people who eat fruit such as oranges tend to eat less at subsequent meals compared to those who ate snacks such as chips, desserts and sweets, etc.)
- Pears (a decrease in overall glucose and cholesterol by eating fruits such as pears and apples)

- Quinoa (offers greater satiety compared to rice and wheat and is therefore an ideal food for fighting obesity)
- Raspberries (reduces glucose levels after starch-rich meals)
- Romaine lettuce (starting off a meal with a low calorie salad gives a sense of fullness and reduced subsequent calorie intake)
- Strawberries (found to control type II diabetes by reducing blood glucose levels after a starchy meal)
- Tea (approx. 10 cups of green tea a day assists in reducing body fat)
- Wheat (a study found that people who consumed the most whole grain foods had a lower BMI. Also lowers total and LDL cholesterol and improves insulin sensitivity)
- Whey protein (gives a sense of satiation and increases skeletal muscle growth better than all proteins).

Eat small meals every 3-4 hours, but when out and about use the following guidelines:
- Make your own food the night before and take it with you so you can avoid fast food outlets
- Carry water and/or diluted juice with you everywhere
- Have fresh fruit, nuts and *healthy* muesli bar snacks available at all times
- Avoid drinking too much tea or coffee because of their diuretic effect
- Include either fresh fruit and/or salad in each meal
- Include a major source of carbohydrates in each meal
- Replace fluids and eat healthy food as soon as possible after your workout.

To work best, everything mentioned in this book needs to be moulded around the following:
- Your specific circumstances
- Your personal and specific needs.

How to start the day

You may have read or heard that some companies are recommending that you wake up and you don't eat for another 5-6 hours. But do we really want to starve ourselves? And won't this lead to overeating late at night? For Wellness FitCoach, it goes against everything related to kick-starting your metabolism with healthy breakfast choices. Lets face it, you need to 'break the fast' in some way, but ultimately if you are not eating a healthy breakfast in the first place, then of course this is not a good way to start the day. The main problem again arises from false advertising.

Breakfast
Kick-start your metabolism by 'Breaking the fast'. So why is breakfast important?
1. After a full night sleep breakfast is vital for helping your metabolic and energy producing processes swing into action
2. Breakfast gives you superior mental performance throughout the morning
3. Breakfast gives you increased physical performance later in the day

4. Food cravings are less likely later in the day, but those who eat a healthier fibre-packed breakfast tend to opt for healthier food choices in the evening
5. When time is short in the morning a healthy cereal is simple to prepare.

Which type?
If you opt for cereals (breakfast in a box) then ultimately you need to read the true content of what you are buying, rather than what's on the front. But generally you are looking for 100% wholegrains with no added sugar or artificial sweeteners/E-numbers and preferably organic. Muesli with natural dried fruit is generally a good choice, which is an oat-based breakfast and normally free from sugar. Skimmed or semi-skimmed milk is fine, but any organic ones such as almond/coconut/rice milk are even better, also water in some cases. Adding your own ingredients such as fresh fruit (chopped banana/apple/blueberries, etc.) and a dash of honey, if you crave a sweet taste, will add fibre and antioxidants to this very important meal.

Extra tips
Muesli can put people off if the consistency is too 'rabbit foody' so if this is the case then use a spoonful of healthy yoghurt instead of the milk. Also, you can soak the muesli in milk overnight and place it in the fridge prior to adding your fruit, etc. in the morning. This option will also save you more time when you awake, and this healthy meal choice can also be used as a snack throughout the day, or even after a workout to promote recovery.

"When you have something for breakfast, you're not going to be starving by lunch."

- Bruce Barton

Lunch
- Add baked beans (protein) to your jacket potato (carbohydrate) and serve with a large green salad (vegetables)
- Try a bean based (legumes) or vegetable soup (homemade)
- Eat a variety of different breads,for example grainy or pumpernickel bread instead of white or wholemeal bread.

Evening meal
- Consider boiled potato or sweet potato instead of mashed potato with your meal
- Choose basmati or easy cook rice
- Include plenty of vegetables with your meals
- Include more beans and lentils in your meal, and try adding them for example in casseroles and curries.

Snacks
- Get into the habit of eating fruit
- Low fat yogurt.

Compulsive eating & food cravings

You can eliminate food cravings by control and eating small amounts of food instead of forbidding yourself food. How do you cope with your repeated cravings of eating treats that will ruin your weight loss attempts? Eating dense low-energy foods like vegetables, fruits and soups as shown by many studies, maintains satiety and reduces energy intake. A more successful weight loss strategy advising individuals in a clinical trial is eating portions of low-energy, dense foods rather than fat reduction coupled with restriction of portion sizes. Satiety can be enhanced and hunger controlled, even restricting energy intake for weight by consuming fulfilling portions of low-energy dense foods. (J.A. Ello-Martin, 2005).

You can do the following things before you 'give in' to unplanned cravings:
1. Have a glass of water or a cup of herbal or fruit tea when you feel like eating i.e. drink something before eating as maybe you were only thirsty and not hungry at all.
2. Do some brisk walking, even if it's to another floor in your office building, remind yourself of your goals whilst undertaking anything physical.
3. So you don't lose that fresh and clean feeling, carry your toothbrush and toothpaste with you everywhere, even if it's just to give you something to do to take your mind off food.
4. Ask yourself if you are actually hungry, and if you still really want the food.
5. Decide on your real temptation after examining the situation. Why did you have a sudden urge to eat something? Was the food visible to you? Did a walk make you pass the fridge? Did boredom strike you with your current activity? You will soon realise that wanting the food was nothing more than an impulse.
6. Think about what will truly satisfy your hunger after judging if you are physically hungry or not. Do you need to eat something crunchy, a bit of sweet, a little something to nibble, or something salty or something more filling? To satisfy any type of hunger, you can always find a healthy alter native. For unhealthy treats, keep healthy substitutes at hand.
7. If everything fails, eat the food. But…enjoy the food you desperately wanted without a guilty conscience, but…eat it slowly. Afterwards exercise a little extra, and have smaller portions throughout the day to compensate for your craving to get things back on track.

Create a new civilisation

Do you find yourself being encouraged to fall back into the easier option of weight loss with a constant reliance and needless crisis for medical support? When you decide to lose weight, you must remember and keep it at the forefront of your mind that you are turning your back on poor health and a life-threatening disease.

When you begin to eat more healthily, admittedly you won't feel better immediate-

ly, and for 3-4 days you may even have some or all of the following symptoms:
- You may feel worse than you did before you started eating more healthily
- You may get a sore throat
- You may even feel anxious
- In reality you will feel fatigued.

But in time you will feel 100% better, with more far-reaching benefits than you can possibly list here. You will most certainly have an increase in vitality and virility, and you will almost definitely reduce your cravings.

Food prescription

In order to avoid the problems that follow from dietary deprivation, we have supplied you with some options to choose from in order for you to feel nourished and satisfied. We have chosen foods that will make you feel full by controlling your hunger, and because they have fewer calories they will assist you in losing weight too.

Eat more fruit and veg
How many times do you hear this? Reason? The water and fibre in such foods provides you with more volume and weight, but less calories. Fruit and vegetables take longer to digest too.

Foods to 'avoid' and 'try'

Avoid	Try
Avoid coffee and croissant for breakfast	Organic cereal/wholegrain oats/muesli and add blueberries to it or organic eggs, omelette, etc.
When you have a snack – avoid unhealthy fast food	Having raw vegetables, nuts, etc. at the ready
Choose your drinks wisely – avoid soda (coke, etc.) and any concentrated fruit juices	Try fresh, frozen or canned fruit (unsweetened)
When you have a main meal – decrease the size of your meat portion	Increasing the vegetable portion
If you have a wholemeal pasta meal – avoid cheesy or meat sauces	Try mixing sautéed vegetables in
Liven up a salad – avoid high calorie dressings	Try asking for it on the side or make your own, add mandarin orange/peach slices, or pineapple and pomegranate
If you eat bread – avoid saturated fats i.e. Margarine	Try any Omega variety (3,6, etc.) and spread sparingly
Check if your carbs are refined – avoid refined grains	Choose wholewheat bread, wholegrain pasta, oatmeal, brown rice, wholegrain cereal, wholegrain rice

Proteins & Dairy – decrease your 'not so good fats' and overall calories	Increase your protein (+fibre) by eating beans, peas, lentils, also grilled fish, skinless white meat (chicken, turkey, etc.). Try egg whites too and search for dairy labelled 'fat free'
Fats – reduce your saturated fats	Try nuts, seeds, flax oil, olive oil and safflower oil and use sparingly
Sweets – avoid having a large serving	Try a small serving of fresh fruit with low fat yogurt, or cookies made with wholewheat flour, or low fat ice cream, or cacao or dark chocolate

♥Task 22

Search for fruit, vegetables and wholegrains and foods labelled low fat with no added sugar or artificial sweeteners/E-numbers. Also lean cut meats, i.e. meat with minimum or no fat on it.

A-Z of choice

Here are some of the best fibre-rich foods for a flat stomach and a full belly.

Fibre-rich Foods		
Apples	Brown Rice	Oatmeal
Artichokes	Brussels Sprouts	Oranges
Arugula	Butter Beans	Peaches
Asparagus	Chick peas	Peas
Avocado	Edamame	Pears
Bananas	Figs	Pinto Beans
Barley	Green Beans	Quinoa
Black Beans	Kidney Beans	Raspberries
Blackberries	Lentils	Red Beans
Blueberries	Lima Beans	Spinach
Black Eye Peas	Mixed Greens	Sweet Potato
Broccoli	Navy Beans	White Beans

So, you've got a lot of choices there ☺ and that's not even an extensive list!

Again, by replacing sugary foods with fibre-rich foods, you'll automatically cut a tremendous amount of calories from your diet while enjoying much more filling and satiating meals...a clear win to keep your belly satisfied and your waistline slim.

A-Z of herbs & spices

Food Types	Why it is a Good Choice For Your Weight Loss & Overall Health:
Cinnamon	Regulates blood sugar, reduces glucose, triglyceride and LDL cholesterol
Cloves	Is the spice that contains the highest amount of antioxidants, can be used as a painkiller, it also eases colds and allergies
Coriander seeds	Anti-inflammatory, fights colon cancer and lowers cholesterol. Provides Vitamin C, phosphorous, potassium, zinc, copper, dietary fibre, calcium & iron!
Cumin	A potent anti-inflammatory & antioxidant that may help stop tumour growth.
Dried Red Pepper	May lower the risk of skin & colon cancers
Garlic	Anti-fungal and anti-bacterial
Ginger	Aids in weight loss and detoxification. Lowers cholesterol, helps increase insulin sensitivity, reduces inflammation, treats arthritis, contains a very large amount of antioxidants, increases circulation and calms digestive problems, decreases motion sickness and nausea
Mustard	Contains anti-cancer compounds
Nutmeg	Contains antibacterial compounds that may help fight listeria, E. coli and salmonella
Oregano	A natural source of omega-3 contains a higher amount of antioxidants than blueberries, rich in vitamin k, iron, and manganese, kills e-coli, salmonella and other food pathogens
Paprika	Anti-inflammatory and antioxidant
Turmeric	Helps reduce obesity and metabolic diseases, it can also eliminate the growth of cancer cells
Rosemary	Fights against obesity and many other medical conditions, rosemary oil can improve cognitive performance and fight off free radicals.

Metabolism

Both green and black teas have been found to give the metabolism a kick and even detoxify harmful chemicals. Studies, including a Japanese report published in 2008, 'Annals of Nutrition and Metabolism', found that those who drank green or black tea lost more weight while lowering 'bad' or LDL cholesterol and increasing 'good' (HDL) cholesterol levels.

Is today's diet linked to depression?

Most humans are now paying the price for the change in agricultural practices and poor eating habits, especially compared with hunter-gatherer cultures of old.
Meat from animals these days (that's not free-range) provides virtually zero omega-3 fats at all, and will usually have a body fat content of around 30%, which is incidentally similar to that of a sedentary human.

Mood foods
Foods to improve your mood include:
- Avocado – have many benefits to help elevate your spirit
- Spinach – nutrient-dense working wonders not only on your mood, but also your health and prevents illness
- Raw cocoa – high in magnesium and triggers the brains production of natural opioids
- Chia seeds – potent vegetarian source of omega 3, and packed full of amino acids
- Sunflower seeds – rich in Vitamin E, selenium and magnesium.

Improve your mood physiologically
In order to assist in the reduction of depressive tendencies do the following:
- Consume more omega-3 fats from eating more fish than meat, and eat plenty of green leafy vegetables
- Choose exercise instead of medication.

EPA/DHA deficiency leads to depression so what can we do about it?
First we must know what it is. Omega-3 fatty acids are a group of three fats: alpha-linolenic acid (ALA), docosahexaenoic acid (DHA), and eicosapentaenoic acid (EPA).

Your diet should provide equal amounts of unsaturated fats from the omega-6 and omega-3 family, and these are both essential fats, with omega-9 that includes fat sources such as olive oil that are not essential but are good for you in very small amounts. Some sources of omega-3 fats include:

- Fish such as fresh tuna, sardines, salmon, mackerel, herring, trout, halibut, oysters, etc.
- Fortified dairy and juices such as milk, fresh juices, eggs (produced by chickens fed omega-3s in their grain), soy milk, yogurt, etc.
- Grains and nuts like wholemeal bread, flour and pasta (not white or bleached brown), healthy cereal like oats, oatmeal, etc., flaxseed, organic peanut butter, pumpkin seeds, walnuts, etc.
- Fresh Produce. In addition to omega-3, green leafy vegetables such as spinach, parsley, brussels sprouts, kale, mint, watercress, etc. are a good source of fibre and antioxidants.

- Oils like cod liver oil, mustard oil, soybean oil, rapeseed oil, walnut oil, flaxseed oil, etc.

"You are setting yourself up for illness and injury if you don't improve your calorie consumption in some way."

- Wellness FitCoach

Protein sources
Approximately 30% protein intake should come from beef, pork, lamb, poultry and game meat (preferably grass not grain fed and free ranging sources). Fish and seafood should also be consumed as part of this intake.

Food Types	Amount of Protein
Spirulina	60%
Spinach	49%
Kale	45%
Barley Grass	45%
Broccoli	45%
Cauliflower	40%
Mushrooms	38%
Sprouts	35%
Parsley	34%
Beef	26%
Cucumber	24%
Chicken	23%
Cabbage	22%
Green Pepper	22%
Chia seeds	22%
Tomatoes	18%
Brazil Nuts	17%
Romaine Lettuce	16%
Eggs	12%
Goji Berries	12% &10% fibre

Saturated vs unsaturated

Unsaturated	Which to eat
Olive oil Sesame oil Nut oils Flaxseed oil	Organic, extra-virgin and cold-presses varieties are best. Ideally consumed without heating.
Avocado Nuts & seeds	Organic & raw is ideal, best eaten soaked or sprouted then re-dried at a very low oven temperature or in a dehydrator.

Saturated	Which to eat
Coconut oil Palm oil	Organic is ideal, great for non-animal based options. These are great for cooking at high temperature.
Butter Ghee Lard Tallow Full-fat dairy Meat & fish with visible fat	Organic, grass-fed/from pasture-raised animals or wild fish is ideal, followed by organic.

Unsaturated	Which to ditch
Canola oil Corn oil Soybean oil Grape seed oil	These all go through extreme processing to produce a high yield.

Saturated	Which to ditch
Margarine Hydrogenated oils Partially-hydrogenated oils Trans-fats Fat from meat that is commercially raised	These are harmful and form molecular structures that do not occur the same way in nature
Butter, Ghee Lard, Tallow Full-fat dairy Meat & fish with visible fat	Organic, grass-fed/from pasture-raised animals or wild fish is ideal, followed by organic.

Superfoods

Superfood	Benefits
Avocado	Good healthy fats that aid in weight loss & burn fat. Prevent & assist arthritis. Reduces & reverses ageing. High in Vitamins A, C, K & B6. Also high in fibre, potassium & folic acid.
Coconut	Accelerates weight loss. Lowers cholesterol. Improves diabetes. Aids digestion. High in protein & calcium & a great natural skin moisturiser.
Lemon	Aids in detoxing & digestion. Burns fat & accelerates weight loss. High in Vitamin C. Relieves constipation & alkalizes the body.
Superfood combination	Benefits
Leafy greens, dried fruit, artichokes or legumes with tomatoes, peppers or citrus	Combining iron-rich foods with those packed with Vitamin C helps your body absorb iron more efficiently.
Green tea & lemon	Adding lemon juice to green tea increases powerful DNA repairing catechins contained in green tea – making the tea five times stronger. Consuming green tea when you eat fish helps block mercury from entering your bloodstream.
Avocados & tomatoes	The monosaturated fat found in avocados boosts the cancer-fighting properties of lycopene found in tomatoes & makes it four times effective.
Dark chocolate & apples	Apples are rich in quercetin – an anti-inflammatory crucial to heart health. Dark chocolate contains powerful antioxidants called flavonoids. This pair forms a tasty snack that fights blood clots, improves circulation & reduces your chances of heart disease.
Bananas & yoghurt	This duo maximises absorption of muscle-repairing glucose & amino acids. After intense exercise, this combination speeds up muscle recovery while strengthening muscle cells.

Jason Vale (2012) is best associated with Juices, and in his book he recommends some really important superfoods such as spirulina, wheatgrass and psyllium husks. Some of their benefits are listed below.

Spirulina
Many people incorporate spirulina into their regular diet as it provides significant health benefits if taken on a daily basis, it also:
- Increases your energy
- Boosts internal cleansing
- Helps with your weight control
- Boosts your body's natural defences.

Wheatgrass
Extensive evidence suggests that if incorporated into your regular diet wheatgrass provides significant health and healing powers.
- The powder preserves all the nutrients and enzymes for everyday vitality and well-being
- It contains over 100 key nutritional elements.

Psyllium Husks
Contain a high level of soluble dietary fibre; therefore, makes you feel full in the stomach which helps with weight loss. They also help with the following:
- Elimination of toxins, chemicals and waste products
- The removal of toxins from the intestines prevents headaches, loss of energy and fatigue
- Doesn't contain gluten, yeast, dairy, sugar, salt or artificial colours or preservatives.

"1lb of fresh wheatgrass is equal in nutritional value to nearly 25lbs of other green vegetables."

- Dr Anne Wigmore

Vitamins and minerals
A diet that is consistently deficient in certain vitamins and minerals will limit your performance.

Vitamins	Optimum Daily Intake	Health Benefits
Vitamin A	1.500mcg	Improves skin & immunity
Vitamin B1 (thiamine)	25mg	Makes energy
Vitamin B2 (riboflavin)	25mg	Makes energy
Vitamin B3 (niacin)	50mg	Lowers cholesterol
Vitamin B5 (pantothenate)	50mg	Improves memory
Vitamin B6 (pyridoxine)	50mg	Balances hormones
Folic acid	200mcg	Protects your DNA
Biotin	50mcg	Vital for children
Vitamin C	1,000mg	Boosts immunity
Vitamin D	5mcg	Builds bones
Vitamin E(d-alpha tocopherol)	100mg	Protects arteries
Minerals	Optimum Daily Intake	Health Benefits

Calcium	200mg	Builds bones
Magnesium	150mg	Keeps you relaxed
Iron	10mg	Carries oxygen
Zinc	10mg	Boosts immunity
Manganese	3mg	Anti-ageing oxidant
Chromium	30mcg	Balances blood sugar

Up-to-date food pyramid

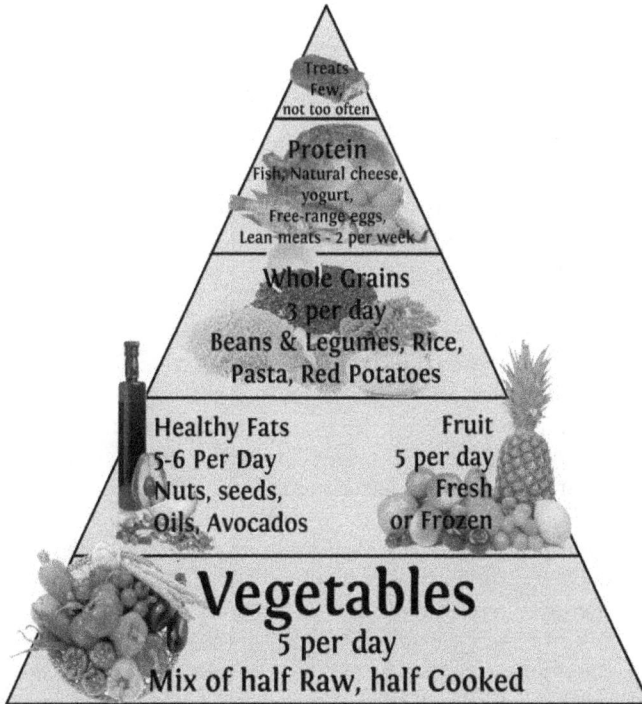

Treats
Few,
not too often

Protein
Fish, Natural cheese,
yogurt,
Free-range eggs,
Lean meats - 2 per week

Whole Grains
3 per day
Beans & Legumes, Rice,
Pasta, Red Potatoes

Healthy Fats
5-6 Per Day
Nuts, seeds,
Oils, Avocados

Fruit
5 per day
Fresh
or Frozen

Vegetables
5 per day
Mix of half Raw, half Cooked

In addition to the content within the above Food Pyramid, be aware of the following:
• Go organic wherever you can
• Take daily supplements (based on your Doctor's recommendations), especially if you are deficient in any area
• Drink herbal teas whenever you can
• Use healthy herbs and spices within your cooking

Andi score

An excellent guide to nutrition is the ANDI score, which stands for 'Aggregate Nutrient Density Index'. An ANDI score shows the nutrient density of a food on a scale from 1 to 1000 based on nutrient content. ANDI scores are calculated by evaluating an extensive range of micronutrients, including vitamins, minerals, phytochemicals and antioxidant capacities. On the website link below you can access the following food types:

- Green Vegetables
- Non-green Vegetables
- Fruit
- Beans
- Nuts and Seeds.

http://www.wholefoodsmarket.com/healthy-eating/health-starts-here/resources-and-tools/top-ten-andi-scores

Lifestyle Challenge Recommendations:
1. Don't discount the role of liquids in your dietary audit because if you are like the majority of people, you may turn to caffeine to jumpstart a sluggish day. What millions don't understand is that it can do more harm than good as it boosts the production of adrenaline, another stress hormone.
2. Dependant on where you are during the day, in the house or at the office, it can get quite stuffy and it's easy to get dehydrated without noticing. If you always have a glass of water and sip it regularly you won't get the urge to be constantly making cups of tea and coffee, which will dehydrate you more and often lead to eating something alongside. Cake and a glass of water are just not the same as cake and coffee.
3. Throw a cup of blueberries in your cereal every morning to get two servings right away, or include two fruits or vegetables in every meal like a salad with mandarin oranges, and then eat another as a snack. In this case, no matter what, you will get at least seven servings a day.
4. With reference to vegetables, you can incorporate produce powder into yogurt, soups and smoothies by adding a powdered vegetable supplement into your morning shake. All these added extras to make it easier are all available at health food stores around the world.
5. Steaming vegetables makes them easier to digest and helps you absorb more nutrients, but just be careful not to overcook them. A good marker is that if the vegetables lose their vibrant color, chances are they've also lost many of their vitamins.
6. Your body has mechanisms for setting your weight where it wants it to be, which can best be described as similar to the way you set the temperature of your house with a thermostat. So the right tool for the job of losing weight is one that changes your body's set point, so you need to change your metabolism.

72

☀️ Re-energise your digestive system

Recommended for you is a 24 hour cleanse to re-energise the digestive system that will sharpen your concentration and focus and improve your sleep patterns. But, more importantly, it will allow nutrients to be better absorbed into your whole body, which will ultimately provide you with more energy:

- Drink the juice of one lemon in fresh water (during the morning hours)
- 10-30 minutes later, consume any fruit or vegetable (juiced yourself) or fresh, raw vegetables in boiling water (soup)
- Water (distilled) should be more than the recommended daily amount, shoot for approximately 10 glasses
- Throughout the 24 hours, you may consume any kinds of vegetables prepared as above, but the fruit should be one serving and just one kind, no combinations
- No salt is to be consumed throughout.

It will vary with each individual, but normally it should take between 1-3 days. You will know how it has gone if you are constantly on the toilet after each meal and if you are not then perhaps you should continue after the 24 hours, but definitely complete the cleanse once or twice a week.

Regardless of the time it takes for your initial cleanse to produce the desired results, going through this cleansing process will become easier and easier in subsequent weeks and your system will become cleaner and healthier as time goes on. Nutrition tips and diet information from different sources often conflict with each other, so you should always check with your doctor first.

♥ Task 23
Lifestyle Challenge 2

- I will attempt to cleanse my body of toxins prior to beginning this program
- I will eat a healthy breakfast to kick-start my metabolism
- I will eat the right foods at the right time and limit my processed foods
- I will eat more than three healthy meals per day in order to lose weight
- I will carry a bottle of water everywhere, drink hot water and lemon or unsweetened iced teas for their anti-aging antioxidants
- I will eat lots of fresh whole fruits and vegetables or make smoothies
- I will eat smaller servings of high fat/high calorie foods or just simply replace them with healthier foods or eat them less often
- I will pay attention, enjoy my food and eat more slowly, not in front of TV, PC or while on Facebook, etc.
- I will not eat fried food or takeaway meals and I will choose my meals at home or at the restaurant more wisely by eating more grilled food, etc.
- I will definitely eat more protein (chicken, turkey and fish) on a daily basis
- I will remember that alcohol has many hidden calories
- I will make my snacks healthier with tuna, chicken salad, etc.

Do not continue until you have written these down or cut them out to keep safe. You are now more than on your way to success.

In order to avoid eating unhealthy food you need to allow time for shopping. For some people this can be torture but it is very important:

- Buying, preparing and eating healthy food.

Task checklist

Part 3: Nutrition
☐ ♥ Task 19
Write down what you definitely know to be true.
☐ ♥ Task 20
Without healthy nutrition, your weight loss is doomed for failure, and because our philosophy does not include negativity we task you with doing the following...
☐ ♥ Task 21
Write down some of your current food choices that you feel could be better.
☐ ♥ Task 22
Search for fruit, vegetables and wholegrains and foods labelled low fat with no added sugar or artificial sweeteners/E-numbers. Also lean cut meats i.e. meat with minimum or no fat on it.
☐ ♥ Task 23
Lifestyle Challenge 2 – nutrition.

Part 4: PHYSICAL

Sticking to an exercise program

People are mostly under the impression that exercise helps them in developing a good physical health. Although very few know that exercise can work wonders when it comes to mental health as well by reducing depression amongst many other benefits.

Sticking to an exercise programme reduces the chance of various diseases such as:
- Cardiac arrests
- Strokes
- Cancers
- Diabetes.

It also lowers blood pressure and assists with improving immunity and bone density.

In 1990, a meta-analysis, which was based on 80 studies of exercise and depression, played an influential role in changing the general notion about exercise. Exercising became the third most viable option after psychotherapy and medication when it comes treating mental disorders.

The research team, which included psychologist Penny McCullagh, PhD, made a few intriguing discoveries:
1. Exercise benefited mental health both immediately and in the long-term
2. Exercising is at its most effective at the start of an exercise program for people who are at their worst physically or mentally
3. Older people benefit more than young in terms of decreasing depression through exercise programs
4. Exercising affects both males and females equally
5. Walking and jogging are the two exercises most extensively researched; however, both aerobic and anaerobic forms helped in treating depression at least to some extent
6. The more people exercised, the greater their chances of coming out of their depressive moods
7. Exercising is at its best when combined with psychotherapy.

Weight can be lost in the long-term by sticking to an exercise program whilst paying attention to the consumption of food in adequate quantities; therefore, burning off excess calories. All of these will help you to maintain a healthy body weight. However, you must realise that the ideal body weight varies from person to person but you have to be realistic and should not always idolise the athletic sportsmen and slim supermodels in your pursuit of losing weight. Workout schedules should be

developed to help you achieve a minimum level of physical fitness, lower cholesterol levels and improve your general health.

IMPORTANT
Your medical practitioner must always be consulted before you start out on an exercise programme, and this approval will become even more necessary if you are
suffering from some kind of prior ailment.

Wellness FitCoach exercise facts

Exercise the mind and body:
1. Exercise increases your metabolism
2. Exercise creates a calorie deficit without triggering starvation mode
3. Exercise helps you sleep better and manage stress better
4. Exercise (strength training) tells your body to keep the muscle, wheras dieting causes muscle loss
5. Exercise increases bone density
6. Exercise helps prevent diabetes, control blood sugar and improve insulin
   sensitivity
7. Exercise improves cardiovascular health
8. Exercise improves mood, helps relieve depression and increases self-
   esteem
9. Exercise increases mobility and quality of life as you get older
10. Exercise helps you keep the weight off long-term.

The power of music
In a series of studies, research has demonstrated that listening to motivational music
before performing an activity is associated with increased strength. Another strategy
that can be used in conjunction with music is video footage. Short motivating video
clips alongside your preferred music can target your ideal psychological state for
improved performance.

Working out to music activates certain pleasure centers in the brain, to not only
make you feel happier, but it may also make you move faster and for a longer period of time which will get you better results on your weight loss journey. The faster
the beat of the music the faster you will move, and therefore your choice of music
can assist you to workout more vigorously.

Do you have time to sit on your backside?

When asked about exercise, 'time' or lack of it is one of the biggest reasons that
people give as to why they don't do it. Yet when asked about sitting in front of the
TV, the internet or playing the PlayStation, time never seems to be an issue.
The main function of your skeleton is to move your body; therefore, the way I see it
is if you don't move you don't function. Without fitness, all the mental stamina in

the world won't help if every muscle in your body is fully exhausted. Exercise is far more cost effective than any other medical drugs such as Prozac, it acts to increase brain serotonin in order to improve your mood and self-confidence.

But does exercise act in the same way? Of course it does.

"Inactivity is not going to help you if you want to lose weight, even if you stand up every hour and generally keep yourself busy can help. It may even prevent you from being in a depressive state."

- Wellness FitCoach

A sedentary lifestyle and lack of physical activity can contribute to, or be a risk for the following:
- Psychological disorders such as anxiety, depression, mood swings
- Cardiovascular diseases like congestive heart failure, hypertension (high blood pressure), coronary heart disease, atherosclerosis
- Weight management – for example, obesity, diabetes, being overweight
- Cancer – Breast, lung, prostate, colon cancer
- Pulmonary diseases like emphysema, chronic bronchitis, asthma
- Musculoskeletal disorders – for example. osteoporosis, osteoarthritis, back pain, bone fractures and connective tissue
- Deep vein thrombosis, lipid disorders, kidney stones
- Mortality rates rise by 30% in elderly men and double the risk in elderly women.

"Move towards your goal, or stay motionless and let it move away from you."

- Your metabolism

No more procrastination

To get what you want you need to learn how to not put things off. When you can see the direct result of your efforts then this provides you with enough encouragement to support you. So the key is to choose the correct programme for you related to your current level.

To get you started
For some people even standing up for a prolonged period is an exercise, but wherever your starting point is the principles are still the same related to good posture, technique, gradual progression, etc. All you need to commit to is any one of the following (or more for better results):
- 10 minutes of your time, 3 times per day

- 15 minutes of your time, 2 times per day
- 30 minutes of your time, 1 time per day.

Ensure you do the following for sustainability:
- *Maintain daily goals* that are progressive and intense enough to get results
- *Plan rewards* for yourself that are relevant to what you have achieved
- *Review your progress* so that you can progress to the next phase
- *Adjust your target goals* if required but keep them realistic and achievable.

Enjoy it

When you find a physical activity that you enjoy doing, your awareness will be so focused you'll find that less effort will be required, because your choice would have made the situation intrinsically rewarding. Regarding physical rewards, Stipek (1996) noted that rewards should be given on the basis of *improvement, effort* and *performance*.

♥ Task 24

Write down some of your current exercise choices that you feel could be better. Examples:
- I don't do any exercise so I could start doing something, even if it is walking after I have eaten
- I currently walk the dogs, so I could start walking faster or even some slow jogging.

Lack of knowledge about the human body

A lack of physical activity is one of the leading causes of preventable death worldwide, but you will be surprised at the amount of people who do not know what's killing them and what will help their body maintain good function. Is it any wonder though by the amount of false advertising and exercise books, etc that tempt you with ways in which you can do this and that in less time?

"The human body has two ends on it: one to create with and one to sit on. Sometimes people get their ends reversed, and when this happens they need a kick in the seat of the pants."

- Theodore Roosevelt

Self-sabotage

Exercising too vigorously in the beginning is the reason a large percentage of new years resolutions and new weight loss/exercise plans fail. However, progressive *non-stressful* exercise can improve the following:
- The immune system
- Reduce the chances of heart disease
- Increase lifespan.

For example: Do something physical by moving a minimum of 3x per week for 30 mins, at 70% of your maximum effort.

"Exercise to stimulate, not to annihilate. The world wasn't formed in a day, and neither were we. Set small goals and build upon them."

- Lee Haney

How important is your health?

According to a 10-year study published in the British Heart Journal, higher levels of physical activity appears to reduce the risk of heart disease by having favourable effects on blood-clotting mechanisms. This echoed similar findings from a number of earlier studies, which had found that exercise tends to decrease the blood's thrombolytic tendency.

Exercise increases High Density Lipoproteins (HDL) i.e. good cholesterol to help prevent blocked arteries. Doctors recommend a 'low fat diet' in order to reduce *total* blood cholesterol, but if this is not combined with exercise there will also be a reduction in HDL (good) cholesterol too.

Therefore:
1. Exercise lowers Low Density Lipoproteins (LDL) i.e. bad cholesterol, and maintains or increases HDL (good) cholesterol, with no risk of reducing it
2. A low-fat and high-carbohydrate diet can increase triglyceride levels (blood fats), but it has been demonstrated that exercise reduces triglyceride concentrations.

IMPORTANT
Exercise must be maintained for at least four months to bring about the beneficial increase in HDL.

"I really believe the only way to stay healthy is to eat properly, get your rest and exercise. If you don't exercise and do the other two, I still don't think it's going to help you that much."

- Mike Ditka

Get active

Fitness is *not* about a look; it's about a feeling. It's also about:
- The high you feel after a great run
- The strength you feel after completing a set of push ups
- The excitement you feel when your jeans fit
- The joy you feel when you receive a compliment from a friend
- How much more healthier you feel afterwards
- To avoid feeling 'low'.

79

The brains endorphin levels are increased too, which gives you that sense of well-being.

"Physical fitness is not only one of the most important keys to a healthy body, it is the basis of dynamic and creative intellectual activity."

- John F. Kennedy

♥Task 25

Without exercise, weight loss is doomed for failure, and because our philosophy does not include negativity, we want to avoid the word 'failure'. We task you with doing one or more of the following:

1. Hire a personal trainer or ask Wellness FitCoach for advice on exercise.
2. Try something new that is instructor-led, something that challenges you but something you feel you will stick with. Buy 21-30 sessions of any exercise programme (yoga, spinning, boxing, personal training, etc.). Why 21-30 you may ask? Because this will firstly make you committed to attending the sessions and secondly it will create a new habit. But more importantly it will assist you with your plan. Also, 21 days is our trademark selling point; therefore, we state 21-30 days here because you may have days off. Whereas with our programme it is 21 days from start to finish with no days off, and this ensures that new habits will be engrained within your mind.
3. Do something different (physically) each day for 30 minutes, for the rest of your life. Something that makes your heart pump faster and makes you feel good afterwards i.e. walking/jogging/running, cycling, push ups, sit ups, stair climbing, etc.

"Success is not the result of spontaneous combustion, you have got to set yourself on fire for it."

- Anonymous

Your lifestyle

How easy is it to walk away from your past and into your future?

To get you started with movement, let us take a look at walking and just a few of its advantages. A walk may be just the thing you need to get you through your day. It can set the stage for inspired thinking and major mental breakthroughs because when you walk, you stimulate portions of the brain in the right and left hemispheres, giving you access to more areas of your brain than when you're sitting still.

A million years of evolution have equipped our bodies to operate in an optimal way when we're walking and its part of our body's normal restorative process. Walking not only lowers your stress levels, it allows you to sleep better, improve your mood and of course it assists your diet regarding weight loss.

80

A few other advantages of walking are:
1.　It is simple
2.　It is cost effective
3.　It is enjoyable
4.　You can walk anywhere
5.　You can walk at anytime
6.　It is low impact
7.　It is easy on your joints
8.　It is easy to fit into your day.

Technique for walking

Believe it or not, there is a technique for walking as there is for all activities of fitness, but it mainly correlates to maintaining the correct posture.

Lift your head
A jutting head or chin can throw your neck and spine out of alignment, which in turn can cause strain. Therefore, you should lengthen the spine and the back of your neck to bring your shoulders to the proper position and allow your spine to unfurl. These pointers should help your body find its natural alignment.

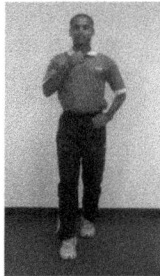

Engage your abdominals
A weak core, which puts excess pressure on the discs between your vertebrae, causes compression in the spine that can result in disc degeneration over time. Therefore, you should gently draw your navel in toward your spine to strengthen and stabilise your core muscles. All of these pointers will help tone abdominals, reduce pressure on your discs and will ultimately safeguard you against back injury. Better alignment of the pelvis, spine and rib cage protects your knees and lets your skeleton support your body more efficiently.

Don't squeeze
Overactive glutes work overtime even when they don't need to and this is often an unconscious attempt to stabilise the body. Clenched buttocks push the thigh bones forward, constricting the hips and lower back. Therefore, you should release the glutes as you walk and let your hips drift back slightly so they can sway naturally.

All of these pointers will help reduce lower back strain and reduce tension. Plus, allow your abs to engage and stabilise the body rather than rely on your glutes to do the work.

<u>Short stride</u>
Over striding, which causes your leg muscles to work too hard, forces the knee into hyperextension that can degrade the joint over time. Focus your energy forward and keep hips, knees and ankles in line by taking narrow, straight steps.

<u>Progressive</u>
Once the correct technique and posture have been mastered, then the pace and/or the distance can be gradually increased for more rapid results. Once your heart rate is increased then the body can become more conditioned. Working out too hard though, may boost inflammation levels rather than reduce them and, while some muscle soreness is warranted, if you're feeling exhausted or overly achy, rest a day before hitting the exercise again. All the walking in the world won't do you any good if you're tweaking your knee, jostling your spine or overtaxing your tight muscles.

While walking, the breathing should be deep, which will ensure that your lungs are being filled in a comfortable manner (during inhalation) and the exhalation should not be forced too much. The best advice is to breathe however you feel comfortable, although it is advised to try and breathe in through the nose and out through the mouth. Once you have been walking for some time and your body has become accustomed to it, then you can include a little jogging. For example, walk, jog and then walk again and it should be logged how far and for how long for each so that you can see your improvements along the way. We have provided you with some progressive programs to work from so that you can choose which one will be more suited to you personally.

IMPORTANT
Even though it's great to have a workout partner, if you find yourself walking and having a nice conversation with your friend, then you can guarantee that you are probably not walking fast enough for the desired results.

How to choose the right location to exercise?

<u>Outdoors</u>
There are many advantages to walking outdoors compared to walking to a DVD or on a treadmill and the same principles apply for running too. Even though running places more stress on your joints, these stresses can be limited greatly if you progress gradually from walking to running over a period of time chosen by you. Choose to walk somewhere soothing, like around a lake, instead of near a busy road and do your best to maintain an easy walking technique. Boost the intensity of your workout by using hills or by walking on grass, sand or trails. To quicken your pace,

bend your arms to 90 degrees and swing them across your body and take quicker steps rather than long strides.

Treadmill
If you're starting out on the treadmill, then 10 to 15 minutes is enough to begin with and the recommended amount is around three times a week. The advantage of the indoor treadmill is that you can also work up to performing upper body exercises holding weights throughout the period of time you are on the treadmill, and of course the advantage to using the incline button to work your leg muscles more.

In the home
If the gym scenario is not right for you and you don't really like the idea of people seeing you walking or running around your neighbourhood, there are certain alternatives. First of all, you could get someone to drop you off a set distance away and pick you up somewhere else. Remember, there is almost always a way around a particular problem or excuse. The choice of many people is to buy a fitness DVD. I remember a client that started to challenge her lifestyle in the New Year who showed me a DVD that she had bought and tried it out and enjoyed it. The workout lasted for approximately 20 minutes. The best part about her motivation and realistic way of thinking was that she already knew that this wouldn't quite be enough but she knew that the DVD also came in 40 and 60 minute versions. You can get out of these DVD workouts what you need and in time your body and mind will tell you when you need to do more. You will either be very bored with doing them or you will get to a point where your results have reached a plateau and you will no longer feel you are progressing.

Our overall point is... at least you are moving, and in some cases more than you were previously but you should continue to progress this over time with what exercise and/or activity you have chosen, until you reach your goal(s).
In the home workouts, you can use the DVD or a treadmill and you should try to implement resistance exercises, which we will explain in more detail later in this chapter. The underlying factor is convenience to you yourself, just as Douglas Brookes, author of *Your Personal Trainer* states "The opportunity to workout needs to be available at every turn in your daily schedule. It makes sense to be committed to exercise in a variety of ways that makes exercise easy, accessible and convenient. At every turn, the chance to agitate your body on a regular basis should be underfoot." In the beginning, whether you are walking, jogging or running, you must keep your pace semi comfortable so that you can maintain it for a long period of time. We call this the active rest phase and you will understand this when I inform you of how low level interval training works. This method will give you a good platform and base to work from, as when it comes to working in short bouts (low level intervals), your body will be aerobically accustomed and will adjust accordingly.

WARNING
The majority of people on new programs start off too fast too soon and therefore

83

can't physically or mentally continue, and eventually they give up. You must remember that everything you change in your lifestyle must be maintained and everything you do must be achievable and progressed accordingly. Giving up in our opinion is not an option!

How does interval training get you quicker results?
Any form of exercise helps but there are ways you can rapidly increase your body's power to burn food calories even when you're sleeping. By alternating periods of intense exercise with slower periods, which is known as interval training, this exercise pattern fine tunes your metabolism. You can choose to walk, jog, cycle, swim or row it's up to you, and it basically consists of exercising for a set time i.e. one minute at almost your maximum capacity and then for another set time i.e. three minutes at a moderate capacity (active rest). You can increase the time at maximum capacity and lower the recovery time (moderate capacity or active rest). Within the next set of challenges we have developed workout programs that can be attempted when the time is right for you.

If you attempt the programs and stick to them and progress them accordingly, then this could be the difference between losing weight long-term or sticking to a diet that will keep you bouncing right back to where you started. The programs we have developed for you are only examples but ultimately, when it comes to setting priorities for yourself, if you choose three intense workouts each week, it will be better than five gentler ones. It's as simple as that and, in actual fact, the more intense workouts will actually take up less time (even though your warm up will need to be slightly longer to reduce the risk of injury). Don't toss the notion of long bouts of cardio out the window, but you should definitely consider adding short bursts of exercise into your day as a challenge. Maybe perform higher intensity intervals once a week. For example, choose a landmark, such as the end of the block, and walk at top speed until you reach it. Repeat this four to eight times on your walk.

Short versus long bouts
As with everything in the health and fitness world, there are arguments for and against anything and everything. But with the debate about short, high intensity workouts versus long ones, the debate has been highlighted by John M Jakicic and colleagues from the *University Of Pittsburgh School Of Medicine* in Pennsylvania, USA. Their results suggested that short bouts of exercise may enhance exercise adherence and weight loss and produce similar changes in cardio-respiratory fitness when compared to long bouts of exercise.

NOTE
Intensity is about getting the most out of your cardio in the least amount of time, so revamp your cardio program with new energising short burst intervals.

Why does building your strength ensure long-term weight loss?
Did you know that you already possess the most powerful fat burner? It's your muscle. So why punish yourself and risk the loss of your fat burning potential? Adding

84

just 10 pounds of muscle to your body will burn off 62 pounds of fat over the next year, even while you are sleeping, and it will continue to do so day after day, week after week, month after month and year after year. Performing cardiovascular exercises at 50% of your maximum heart rate for a minimum of an hour was always the preferred option for a personal trainer to tell his clients and, in some cases, that is true.

But what gets better and quicker results for weight loss? In 2006, Stiegler, from sports medicine, suggested from his research that "strength training may have greater implications than initially proposed for decreasing body fat and sustaining fat free mass. Also, adding exercise programs to dietary restriction can promote more favourable changes in body composition than diet or physical activity on its own."

Strength training has the following benefits:
- Strength training builds muscle
- Strength training turns your body into a more effective calorie burner
- Strength training helps prevent osteoporosis
- Muscle burns fat
- Muscle is more metabolically active than fat.

Just to reiterate what you read earlier, if you don't want to go to the gym and you want to avoid intimidating situations by doing certain things at home, keep a set of weights in an accessible place at home for when you do your walking routine to a DVD or on your treadmill.

Resistant to resistance training
Toned simply means you have shed the fat that once covered your muscles and you can see your muscle definition which gives your body a lean, tight shape. The only reason some women feel like they look bulky is because they have excess body fat whilst building muscle and they are simply not eating in a way that supports fat loss.

You won't bulk up
Facts:
- If you are female, you won't end up looking like a man
- Women simply do not have enough testosterone to get big and bulky
- You will achieve a lean, toned and firm body if you do regular resistance exercises.

Realisation
Now you can start to realise what your body has to offer you. Your body is the answer to the results you require, why do you think yoga has been around for so many years? This is because it works. Try practicing some strength training yoga moves, such as maintaining the plank pose, which is similar to holding yourself up during a full body push up. The plank pose not only makes your arms stronger, but it also works your back, abs, and legs at the same time and it is something you could do absolutely anywhere. All of the recommended exercises that are within this book

have an easier alternative way of performing the exercise and, of course, a harder version too. Lean, toned, fit bodies have low body fat and a lot of lean muscle because strength training maintains and increases your muscle mass and decreases your percentage of body fat.

Targeting certain areas
Most of us have someone we admire or look up to, but don't think for one moment that the toned arms or fabulous abs of a celebrity are created by some 'magic' exercise that mysteriously melts fat off a particular area of the body or that they are any more happier with their bodies than anyone else. Now is the time to banish that myth once and for all.

1. There is simply no exercise that acts like a magic eraser to rid your body parts of unsightly fat, as that is not how the body works
2. If you want to lose fat, you need to challenge all of the muscles in your body to boost your metabolism so that you lose fat all over.

Time saver
When it comes to fat loss, isolated shaping exercises are generally a waste of your time, and just because you feel the burn does not mean that you are burning the fat. One of the most effective ways in which to maximise your fat burning potential is through full body, short burst resistance training. By working several muscle groups at once, short burst resistance training has the following advantages:
- Saves time
- Skyrockets your energy levels
- Incinerates fat and calories.

Strength or aerobic training?
You should realise by now that you cannot achieve permanent weight loss with just dieting alone. Your choices are as follows:
- Diet plus strength training
- Diet plus aerobic training
- Diet, strength and aerobic training - advised for more rapid results.

The level of intensity during your workout will dictate which choice will work best for you and the method will have to be convenient to your daily life. You should now be in more agreement that exercise should be an extremely important part of your life and in some respects it is a must if you want rapid results.

Exercises & the right mix

The specific challenges and progressive exercise programs that follow will ensure that your routine is well-rounded, incorporating interval training (workouts of varying intensities) for at least three times weekly and performing a minimum of 20 minutes of strength training (using your own bodyweight) two or three days a week. The intensity level will ultimately depend on where you are at now and what you will be comfortable with. Being realistic is the key to choosing where you start, we

86

can only give you the choices, but please remember one thing, if you push yourself too fast, too soon, you will get despondent and you will more than likely give up, which is not an option!

What simple, easy-to-follow adaptations will get you rapid results?
Talk to your family doctor before you begin any type of exercise program.

PLAN A:
Your doctor can help you determine which exercise program is right for you:
• Walking outdoors
• Walking on the treadmill
• In your home to a walking keep fit DVD.

All of the above choices should be for a minimum of 20 minutes, at least three times a week or more. If your mind and body allows you to, you can incorporate some jogging with your walking routine for faster results, although this is your choice depending on your fitness level. If you choose to walk only, by the end of the 21 days (non-stop) you should be able to walk for 60 minutes non-stop. Whether you choose to just walk or walk and jog, you should build up to incorporate different ratios. For example, '1 in 3' is equal to one minute faster walking or jogging and three minutes of active rest walking. Of course '1 in 3' can also mean 20 seconds of short burst work to 60 seconds of active rest walking or even two minutes to six minutes. We are sure you get the point. As your heart gets accustomed to what you are doing, challenge yourself further by changing the ratio yet again to '1 in 2' or '1 in 1', which basically limits your active rest time and you can ultimately keep increasing your short bursts as much as you can to sustain them.

IMPORTANT
Whenever you active rest walk, you must walk with purpose as if you are late for an appointment. We have termed it as active rest walking because it must be a speed that you can maintain for a long period of time. Never forget the warm up and cool down phases that involve stretching.

PLAN B:
Your doctor can help you determine which exercise program is right for you:
• In a gymnasium
• In your home.
The most important aspects of these plans is good form i.e. engaging your abdominals throughout all movements as much as you can, also breathing correctly and maintaining good posture throughout the duration. It's better to perform good repetitions with strict body positions rather than rushing into something. Each time you try the exercises you will improve your technique over a period of time, and practice does make perfect. Don't forget the warm up and cool down phases that involve stretching.

87

<u>Resistance</u>
As you are already aware, by working several muscle groups at once, short burst resistance training:
- Saves time
- Skyrockets your energy levels
- Incinerates fat and calories.

A table below that briefly outlines the exercises:

Groups	Exercises	Time	Remarks
Ex 1a - c	Plank	Maximum hold in 2 mins	Keep the back straight at all times
Ex 2a - c	Sit-Ups	Maximum in 2 mins	Keep the knees bent at all times
Ex 3a - c	Leg Squat	Maximum in 2 mins	Make sure the knees don't go over the toes
Ex 4a - c	Push-Ups	Maximum in 2 mins	Ensure the hands are in line with shoulders
Ex 5a - c	Stair Step-Ups	Maximum in 2 mins	Stand up with a straight leg every time

You should attempt to complete 2 minutes of work on each exercise, even if you have to stop and carry on. Exercise 1a will be easier than 1b and so on, and your aim should be to hold good form and maintain good posture.

Exercise 1: Plank pose progressions

<u>Exercise 1a</u>

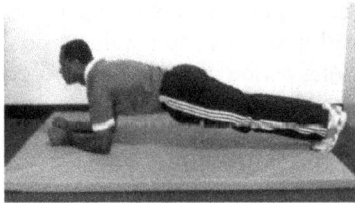

Hold your bodyweight by resting your forearms on the floor.

Exercise 1b

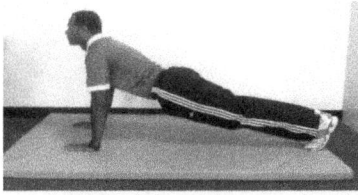

Hold your bodyweight up by your hands and feet.

Exercise 1c

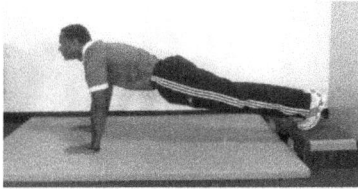

Elevate your feet on a platform to make it more difficult. Attempt this exercise on your forearms if it's too difficult or simply mix it up for variety, just ensure you maintain good form at all times. Start in an outstretched position as in all of the pictures:

- Your hands or elbows should be directly underneath your shoulders
- Your feet should be together
- Keep your back as flat as possible
- Your head and neck should be in line with your spine and you should be looking at the ground slightly in front of you
- Relax the tension from your shoulders.

Aim – To stay in this position as long as possible, just count those seconds and record your achievements in your workout diary!
Tips and techniques – Remember to breathe, pull your belly button into your spine for maximum body tension, and try not to let your hips drop or your buttocks to be raised too high.

Exercise 2: Sit-up progressions

All exercises start off by lying on your back with your knees bent and your feet flat on the floor.

Exercise 2a – start/finish position

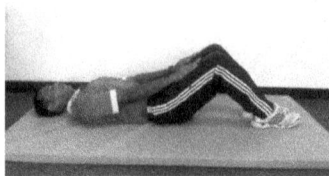

Exercise 2a

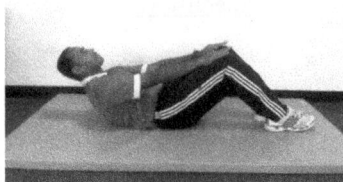

Exercise 2a - Touch the knees with the hands, hold for 2-3 seconds and return to the start.

Exercise 2b

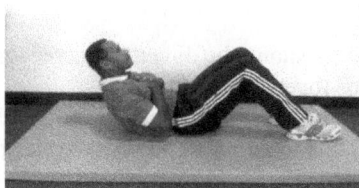

Exercise 2b – Keeping your elbows close in to the chest and your lower back on the floor, curl up so that only your shoulders and upper back come off the ground. Hold again for 2-3 seconds and return to the start.

Exercise 2c

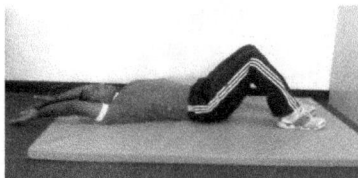

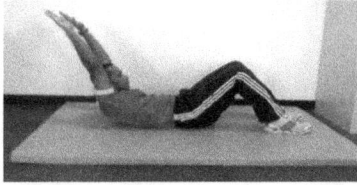

Exercise 2c

Exercise 2c - Extend your arms overhead, slowly raise your arms, head, shoulders, and upper back approx. 30 degrees off the floor. Hold before slowly lowering. Keep your arms straight by your ears and in line with your head. Do not throw them forwards to help you. Add a weighted object in your hands in order to make it more difficult.

NOTE

To maximise *all* exercises, especially the abdominal ones, you can maximise the abdominal pressure by pulling in the stomach as if you are zipping up the fly on an extra tight pair of jeans. If you hold your stomach in whilst breathing out, keep sucking in the stomach more and more as you are breathing out.

You will feel your abdominals and lower back muscles contracting together and, in time, this will improve the support for your spine and lower back. This technique can be done anywhere, even while standing in a queue or sitting in your car. It should especially be utilised during exercise to accompany your body's postural alignment.

Exercise 3: Leg squat

Exercise 3a

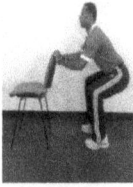

Exercise 3b

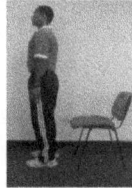

Exercise 3c

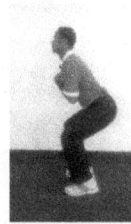

All of these exercises will tone the muscles in the back and front of your thighs and buttocks.

- You should stand with your feet approximately shoulder width apart, your arms either holding an object or fully extended in front of you for balance. Your toes slightly pointing outwards.
- Keep your back straight and squat down until the tops of your thighs are almost parallel to the floor at 90-degrees. Be sure to keep your weight firmly over your heels.
- Rise back to the standing position, making sure that most of your body-weight is through your heels. The chair or alternative object should only be used as a guide. Exercise 3c involves a heel raise at the end of the squat and can be performed without a chair as long as you squat down to a 90-degree angle.

NOTE

As with any exercise, you can progress it accordingly, especially the balance aspect, as it can be progressed by placing your arms across your chest and even closing your eyes, but remember to be safe. You can also add weights to your program by way of dumbbells or a barbell to improve your strength further. Make sure that your knees stay level or behind the toes at all times.

Exercise 4: Push-Up Progressions

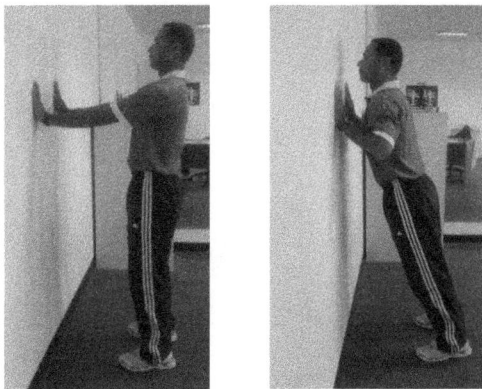

- Ensure the hands are in line with the shoulders and there is a straight line from your head, shoulders, hips and knees, tense the abdominals
- Lower your body slowly towards the wall
- Bend your arms and keep your palms in a fixed position
- Your upper chest should be close to your hands
- Straighten your arms as you push your body away from the wall
- Relax the tension from your shoulders.

Try not to bend or arch your upper or lower back as you push up.

Exercise 4b

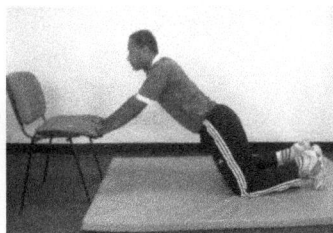

Utilise anything that is elevated off the floor, like a chair against a wall, your bed, your sofa or even your kitchen table, so long as it is secure, flat (level) and stable. You will be testing your body strength more the closer it is to the ground.

- Ensure the hands are in line with the shoulders and there is a straight line from your head, shoulders, hips and knees
- Keep the knees resting on the floor and keep your body straight, lower your body slowly towards the elevated object

- Relax the tension from your shoulders, and bend your arms and keep your palms in a fixed position, then straighten your arms as you push your body up off the object.

Try not to bend or arch your upper or lower back as you push up.

Exercise 4c

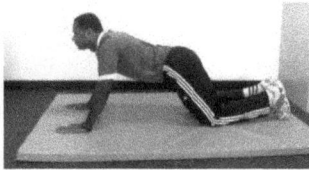

The push-up exercise has been gradually progressed against gravity and now you will be using the floor but still resting the knees. Try it without resting them if you can.

- Ensure the hands are in line with the shoulders and there is a straight line from your head, shoulders, hips and knees
- Relax the tension from your shoulders
- Keep the knees resting on the floor and keep your body straight
- Lower your body slowly towards the floor
- Bend your arms and keep your palms in a fixed position
- Then straighten your arms as you push your body up off the floor.

Try not to bend or arch your upper or lower back as you push up.

Exercise 5: Step-Ups

You can find stairs almost anywhere so make sure you do these exercises. In some ways step ups can be better for you than normal walking to get results quicker.

Exercise 5a

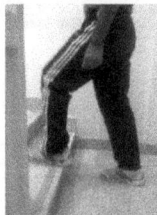

Exercise 5a is a simple step up and step down, changing the legs accordingly. Make sure you step up and straighten each leg fully, carry weights to make harder.

94

Exercise 5b

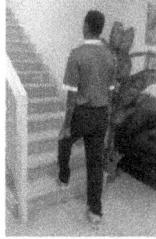

Exercise 5b is a simple walk up the stairs. Turn around at the top and return to the bottom, remembering to straighten the legs fully on each step. Carry weights to make this exercise harder

Exercise 5c

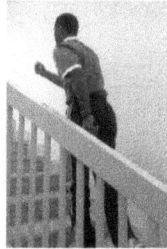

Exercise 5c is a simple jog up the stairs or you can alternate the jog with a walk up the stairs. Try and return to the bottom by walking backwards but remember to be extra safe. You are working your balance and muscles a lot more whilst walking backwards. Instead of walking backwards you can quite simply jog up and down for safety purposes. Carry weights to make this exercise more difficult.

Are you a complete Beginner?…if so try this!

Walking only program for 21 days (continuous)
A daily/weekly walking log should always be kept for motivation and to ensure that you stick to your goals for the new you. Below is an example of a walking only workout program for 21 days that will get yourself focused on your new daily routine, whether it is outside or on a treadmill. If you choose to walk to a DVD for 20 minutes, try and do it once a day at the start of the program, twice a day in the middle and then attempt three times a day nearer the end. This of course depends on the DVD and whether it includes resistance exercises or whether or not the time of the workout is longer than 20 minutes. It's a good idea to get a bunch of DVD's that progress from 20 minutes to 40 minutes and then to an hour.

Day	Date	Distance	Time	Remarks on the walking only program
1	Jan 1	To local shops	20 mins	Today I had to really focus on my posture
2	Jan 2			
3	Jan 3	On treadmill	20 mins	Today I had to really focus on my technique
4	Jan 4			
5	Jan 5	DVD	20 mins	My stretches are now becoming easier
6	Jan 6			
7	Jan 7	Around park	30 mins	Started to walk with more determination today
8	Jan 8			
9	Jan 9	On treadmill	30 mins	Felt good walking today
10	Jan 10			
11	Jan 11	Around park	30 mins	My flexibility is improving
12	Jan 12			
13	Jan 13	20 mins out & back	40 mins	Today I emphasised swinging my arms across my chest
14	Jan 14			
15	Jan 15	DVD	40 mins	20 mins in the morning then in the evening
16	Jan 16			
17	Jan 17	25 mins out & back	50 mins	My posture and technique has now been perfected
18	Jan 18			
19	Jan 19	On treadmill	50 mins	I feel so much more supple
20	Jan 20			
21	Jan 21	30 mins out & back	60 mins	Felt good for achieving my goal

I realise that it states a set time out and the same time back on days 13, 17 and 21. Although this is an example, you should endeavour to walk back at a faster pace because generally you would be warmer and more motivated on the return phase. Walking every other day will give you ample recovery time and you should look forward to the rest time. Ultimately, you will be more than ready for the next workout day. If your day dictates that you cannot workout on a particular day, you can walk on two consecutive days to make up for it.

Remember: This is a challenge for those of you who are complete beginners to exercise, and if this is where you are choosing to begin challenging your lifestyle, then you will be well on your way to changing your life for the better. Out with the old and in with the new.

Have you dabbled before?...if so try this!

Diet, aerobic and strength program for 21 days (continuous)
A daily, weekly aerobic and strength log should always be kept to motivate yourself and ensure that you stick to your goals for the new you. Below is an example of a walking, jogging and strength program for 21 days, to get yourself focused on your new daily routine. The aerobic work can be performed outside or on a treadmill but again, if you choose to walk to a DVD, try to increase the intensity accordingly to encompass the program.

Day	Date	Workout	Time	Remarks on aerobic & strength work combined
1	Jan 1	Walk	30 minutes	Felt good just walking today
2	Jan 2	Strength	20 minutes	Today I concentrated on technique for exercises 1a, 2a, 3a, 4a & 5a
3	Jan 3	**Rest**		
4	Jan 4	Walk	45 minutes	Today I walked very fast for 1 min and 3 mins briskly
5	Jan 5	Strength	20 minutes	I can now do more repetitions of exercises 1a, 2a, 3a, 4a & 5a
6	Jan 6	**Rest**		
7	Jan 7	Walk	40 minutes	Today I walked very fast for 1 min and 2 mins briskly
8	Jan 8	Strength	20 minutes	I concentrated on technique for exercises 1a, 2a, 3a, 4a & 5a
9	Jan 9	**Rest**		
10	Jan 10	Walk	30 minutes	Today I walked very fast for 1 min and 1 min briskly
11	Jan 11	Strength	20 minutes	I can now do more repetitions of exercises 1a, 2a, 3a, 4a & 5a
12	Jan 12	**Rest**		
13	Jan 13	Walk & Jog	45 minutes	Today I jogged for 1min and walked 3 mins briskly
14	Jan 14	Strength	20 minutes	My posture/technique are now fine tuned for all exercises
15	Jan 15	**Rest**		
16	Jan 16	Walk & Jog	40 minutes	Today I jogged for 1 min and walked 2 mins briskly
17	Jan 17	Strength	20 minutes	I feel so much more confident with strength training now
18	Jan 18	**Rest**		
19	Jan 19	Walk & Jog	**30 minutes**	Today I jogged for 1 min and walked 1 min briskly
20	Jan 20	Strength	**20 minutes**	I can feel that my body is now one unit and I look fabulous
21	Jan 21	**Rest**		

Remember: This challenge is for you if you have tried exercise before or you just realise that the strength (fat burning) exercises will get you faster results, and if this is where you are choosing to begin challenging your lifestyle then you will be closer than before to changing your life for the better. Out with the negative thoughts and in with positive ones.

Are you accustomed To Diet, Aerobic & Strength Work Together?

A daily, weekly aerobic and strength log should always be kept to motivate and ensure that you stick to your goals for the new you. Overleaf is an example of a walking, jogging and strength program for 21 days to get yourself focused on your new daily routine.

The aerobic work should be performed outside or on a treadmill, and at this level you shouldn't really be choosing to exercise to a DVD, but if you do, try to increase the intensity accordingly to encompass the program.

Day	Date	Workout	Time	Remarks on aerobic & strength work combined
1	Jan 1	Walk & Jog	30 mins	Today I jogged for 1min and walked 2 min briskly
2	Jan 2	Strength	30 mins	Concentrate on exercises1b+c, 2b+c, 3b+c, 4b+c, 5b+5c
3	Jan 3	Rest		
4	Jan 4	Walk & Strength	50 mins	30 mins fast walk & all exercises 1b-5b
5	Jan 5	Jog	30 mins	30 mins continuous fast jog (include ratios)
6	Jan 6	Strength	30 mins	Posture/technique are now fine tuned for all exercises 1c-5c
7	Jan 7	Rest		
8	Jan 8	Walk & Strength	50 mins	30 mins fast walk & all exercises 1b, 2b, 3b, 4b & 5b
9	Jan 9	Jog	40 mins	40 mins continuous fast jog (include ratios)
10	Jan 10	Strength	30 mins	Posture/technique are now fine tuned for all exercises 1c-5c
11	Jan 11	Walk	45 mins	45 mins continuous fast walk (include ratios)
12	Jan 12	Rest		
13	Jan 13	Jog & Strength	50 mins	30 mins continuous fast jog & all exercises 1b – 5b
14	Jan 14	Walk	60 mins	45 mins continuous fast walk (include ratios)
15	Jan 15	Strength	30 mins	My repetitions and sets are now high for all exercises 1c - 5c

16	Jan 16	Jog	30 mins	30 mins continuous fast jog (include ratios)
17	Jan 17	Walk & Strength	60 mins	30 mins fast walk & all exercises 1c – 5c
18	Jan 18	Jog	40 mins	30 mins continuous fast jog (include ratios)
19	Jan 19	Rest		
20	Jan 20	Walk & Strength	60 mins	30 minutes of each incorporating all exercises 1b – 5b
21	Jan 21	Jog & Strength	60 mins	30 minutes of each incorporating all exercises 1c – 5c

If you think that walking is too easy for you and the rest periods are too often, then you can change them all around to fit in more jogging/running. But you should definitely try and rest in between strength sessions. Try not to have two strength sessions on consecutive days. For example, there are two on days 20 and 21 but we have put that in because there is no strength for two days prior to that. You can of course make one of them an upper body workout and the other a lower body workout for recovery purposes. As mentioned before, these are all examples of how you can implement walking, jogging and strength in a single program.

The allocated 20 minutes for strength can be increased and ultimately all timings can too. But this is why we have included the rest periods to make it more realistic as the rest time is very important so that your body can repair and grow accordingly and more importantly, so that your body can burn fat. Your aim after this challenge should be to implement a good hour a day to your exercise time and if possible, complete a good five days a week with two rest days in between which will be dictated around your weekly plans. When it mentions to include ratios, this can be your choice i.e. you can choose 1 in 1, 1 in 2, or 1 in 3 depending on how you feel on that particular day.

The 20 minutes strength is pure work time and does not include the warm up, stretching or cool down but it's not bad to think that just by going through the exercise program twice you will be activating your fat burning muscles for only 20 minutes (actual work time).

Physiologically, you should complete the strength work prior to the aerobic work because large amounts of energy from the whole body can be expended while walking, jogging or running. Most of the bodyweight exercises are specific to local muscular endurance and will only use up energy from those specific target areas. You should experiment and find out how you feel by performing aerobic first and then strength and vice-versa. It will ultimately depend on your intensity levels and how hard you work whilst walking, jogging or running and this will dictate how you feel when completing the strength work. Also, because some of the exercises we have chosen are specific to core strength, it is sometimes best to perform these at the end of a workout. Fine tune to your specific needs by how you feel. These observations should all be recorded in your diary, which you will need to keep, so that you can look back at your performance on how you felt.

Remember: This challenge is for you if you have tried exercise before or you just realise that the more difficult strength and fat burning exercises will get you faster results, and you will be closer than before to changing your life for the better. Out with the negative thoughts and in with positive ones.

♥Task 26
Lifestyle Challenge 3
I sign to say I agree with the following...
- I will make time for exercising within my daily routine
- I will definitely get up and move around more during the day
- I will walk anywhere I possibly can, avoiding using lifts or escalators
- I can begin to walk slowly and gradually progress to walking faster and further
- I can walk anywhere, whether it be at home on treadmill or to a DVD, or outside
- When I walk faster I will walk with conviction as if I am late for an interview
- In time my body will know when I am ready to alternate walking and jogging
- When I have tried ratio training and I reduce my recovery time I can jog further
- I now know my own body can burn fat so I need to do the exercises in the book
- I will attempt the exercises because they are easy to do and then progress in time.

Even if exercising seems hard, it will become easier as I become more positive.

NOTE
Do not continue until you have written these down or cut them out to keep safe. You are now more than on your way to success, you're almost there.

Rest & recovery

Relax
Rest is an extremely important aspect of your day, and it will be beneficial for you if you can plan for it on a day-to-day basis. We always fit rest periods into an exercise program, so fitting rest into your day should not be missed out on. Even if its 10mins stretching your legs away from the PC at work, or as a rest from the kids at home. The best kind of rest is by way of a silent meditation in solitude i.e. no distractions just peace and quiet. Even if they are not planned, any timeout whatsoever will help you to recharge your batteries at any given time.

💡 Write down where in your day you can fit in a minimum of 10 minutes rest.

Task checklist

Part 4: Physical

☐ ♥ Task 24
Write down some of your current exercise choices that you feel could be better.
☐ ♥ Task 25
Without exercise, weight loss is doomed for failure, and because our philosophy does not include negativity we task you with doing one or more of the following…
☐ ♥ Task 26
Lifestyle Challenge 3 – physical activity.

Part 5: COMBINING IT ALL

Establish where you are currently at

- Do you know what your root cause is/was?
- Have you rid yourself of fear of failure and doubt?
- Do you now have more self-confidence & positivity?
- Can you now control your emotions by having more emotional intelligence?
- How's your fight with depression?

Your emotional intelligence

If you can recognise your different emotional states, assess their effects on your behaviour and manage certain situations by switching your emotional state. This will then provide you with profound results for your weight loss success. To acquire psychological skills such as imagery, goal setting and positive self-talk you will have to get mentally tough, and in time who knows? You may even begin to find exercise enjoyable too. Emotional intelligence is defined as 'the capacity to recognise and utilise emotional states to change intentions and behaviour'. (Mood and human performance: Conceptual, Measurement and Applied issues, 2006).

Move intention into actual behaviour

If you tend to dwell on a negative past then this can only have a detrimental effect on your future outcome, and Biddle and Mutrie (2008) suggest that we should focus more on the action and less on the problem. If you were to analyse any problem all that you will see is negativity in its purest form. So with that in mind, if you try and think in a more positive manner then you are halfway to preventing a problem occurring in the first place.

Regarding your intention to losing weight, taking positive action for better health is the key to your future success.

'Intention-behavior' gap

So now you can focus on how your intentions relate to your actual behaviour.

Look at your environment(s) i.e. your home, your workplace or anywhere you spend your time throughout an average day.

1. How would you say your environment influences your *intention* to lose weight?

Your answer needs to include 'how you think your *current behaviour* about eating healthily and exercising more is affected by your environment?'

2. Think of a strategy you can use to influence your intentions in order to move intention into actual behavior.

Your answer needs to include 'how you think you can change your dialogue (your self-talk) in order to support your desires and what positive words you could use?' One thing is for sure is that there are too many positive psychological benefits when you're healthy. Focussing on exercise in particular, apart from reducing your risk of illness some of the other benefits are listed below.

Exercise adherence *increases* your:
*   Confidence
*   Control
*   Self-esteem
*   Social opportunities.

Exercise and nutrition adherence *improves* your:
*   Mood
*   Cognitive function
*   Quality of life.

Your mind is the key to good thinking, so being fit and strong promotes flexibility of mind and provides you with energy to help you concentrate. Always remember that your brain needs as much care and fine-tuning as your body, especially if you want it to work well for you throughout the whole day.

Moderation & justification are paramount

Food and drink is meant to be enjoyed. Of course you must have the occasional treat, but to deny yourself of the things you like the most will only make you want them more. The solution is to allow yourself those things, but only as a treat i.e. by way of a reward for accomplishing one of your short-term goals, and even then you may have to make up for it later depending on what it was that you had. Your reward doesn't have to be a food type of treat. Surely it is better to be something that is useful to you. For example, perhaps something that you have always wanted?

Choose wisely.

"Those who make the wrong decisions or choices in their lives, will always find an excuse to justify why they did it."

- Wellness FitCoach

Keep it simple
Just as thinking impacts your physiology, your physiology also impacts your thinking. So when you are stressed your brain becomes starved of blood and oxygen. Breathing, exercise and meditation can all assist you in managing these physiological changes. Your brain impacts every area of your body so you need to continuously balance your emotions, and commit to daily self-development, which will assist you with your life, work and your overall health.

Create realistic and manageable rules about what, when and how much you should eat and do physically, also control of your thoughts and viewpoints therefore adding nothing but respect and value to your body. Eating and exercising should be a source of pleasure, eat slowly and train progressively, but remember it should feel really good to nourish and sculpt your body. Learn to know how much food and exercise you genuinely need, listen to your body more and understand that there should be no restrictions when you choose good 'quality' nutrition and exercise.

Nutrition example:
- Lean protein, Vegetables, Fruits, Slow-digesting high-fibre carbohydrates.

Exercise example:
- Endurance based activities i.e. continuous 'steady state' cardio / high repetition, low resistant type functional exercises (controlled speed to master technique but with minimum rest)
- Strength and power based activities i.e. High Intensity Interval Training (HIIT) / low repetition, high resistant type functional exercises (slow tempo/or at speed but with additional rest).

Add physical activity
The good news is that more activity means more 'quality' food, so long as you maintain a balance between the amounts you eat to the level of activity you have achieved.

IMPORTANT
Some key points that most people forget when they train hard is that they feel that they can eat like a race horse, but you still have to take into consideration the *stage of life you are at* and your *'actual' daily needs*.

Psychologically most people go off track at the weekends, so just be aware that this could knock you off track or set you back.
- The rules of the weight loss game should be *your rules* and no one else's
- You should maintain *self-control* from the start
- Without fail you should *remain positive* at all times.

Temptation

Researchers from Duke University, the University of Southern California and the University of Pennsylvania discovered what can resist temptation in college students by asking them about their vices and therefore making them completely conscious and aware of them. The researchers said: "We demonstrate that asking consumers to report their expectations regarding how often they will perform a vice behaviour increases the incidence of these behaviours." It is difficult to resist temptation if one thinks about that which he is trying to resist. The study participants thought of succumbing, so inevitably they did and the main reason why resisting temptation was so difficult for them was actually their own thought processes.

How do you start resisting temptation?

The best way to resist temptation is to turn temptation around. For example, it is better to start eating fresh fruits and vegetables or going out to walk or jog instead of thinking about eating chocolate chip cookies. In comparison, instead of thinking about gambling it is better to focus on the other ways in which the money can be spent. These alternate ways eventually help in resisting temptation. Instead of surfing the net late at night and interrupting your sleep cycle, it is always better to think about the benefits of good sleep or spending quality time with family and friends.

With time you will learn more about resisting temptation and the easier it would be. Rewarding yourself is one wonderful option of resisting temptation; you can bribe yourself with a movie, or a trip to the beach or watching a play or a performance once you are able to resist temptation. There should be an internal focus of control that you need in order to empower yourself.

Resisting temptation whilst shopping

Research shows us that the more somebody talks about a product, the more chances the consumer buys that product. Even harmless questions about that product will lessen the resistance to temptation. In other words the products that people would not normally buy, they would end up buying if the product is talked about. This is how the law of attraction works and the thoughts of the consumers are translated into action. It goes without saying that these were even more evident in people who had less self-control.

What's the pay-off in succumbing to temptation? Is there a benefit in resisting temptation? There is certainly some kind of benefit that you would get for resisting temptation; otherwise nobody would go for that. At the same time it is true that to resist eating a whole packet of biscuits is not half as satisfying as eating them. Eating them would allow you to avoid the otherwise apparent feelings like sadness, disappointment, or loss. In a similar fashion, to resist drinking to excess is not satisfactory, while drinking will help to forget childhood traumatic experiences, it also helps to deal with pain, or even to suppress feelings of shame or guilt. The shift of focus to a form of physical pain also diverts that from the inner emotional turmoil, but behind each and every action we take, there is some reason, even if that reason is not very apparent.

What is advisable is that when you are struggling with temptation, you should try to look beyond the situation and see what the ultimate result is behind succumbing to temptation or resisting temptation. It should be kept in mind that resisting temptation would eventually lead to a happy and healthy life.

Willpower

As you can appreciate, the maximum length of time that people last with their new years resolutions is approximately two-three months. In most cases people just think it's a good idea because everyone else seems to be doing it, and they don't really plan what they are going to do or set any realistic goals. Consequently, their willpower to stop eating and drinking too much of the wrong things reduces so much so, that the actual resolution begins to feel like a totally bad idea in the first place.

Roy Baumeister and John Tierney (2011) quite rightly point out though that 'being overweight is not a telltale sign of weak willpower, even if most people think so.' So how do you last the distance in order to achieve permanent weight loss success? As you are now discovering, it's a total mind-body combination but it's not rocket science is it? Baumeister and Tierney continue to explain that, 'you must use self-control to make gradual changes that will produce lasting effects, and you have to be especially careful in your strategies.'

As you can appreciate you are going to face certain challenges at every stage of the self-control process:
- From setting your goal
- To monitoring yourself on a daily basis
- To strengthening your willpower.

The above processes revert back to good old-fashioned planning, preparation and forward thinking, and therefore if you have a strategy (planned in advance) for the inevitable temptations, then this in itself will give you enormous confidence and should maintain your motivation throughout.

Dr Cummins (2012) says it best – Don't put yourself in temptations way, or if you do, have a plan.

She wrote an interesting article about her own particular experience within her own family home: She first of all mentions that she didn't really care too much for most types of candy, but she does admit that like most women, chocolate was a different matter, but she didn't keep it in her house at all. When her children brought home trick or treat candy, her husband was under strict orders to hide the chocolate where she could not find it. Her side of the contract was not to look or ask for it. Knowing her weakness, she enacted a plan and it has worked for her for years.

106

In Dr Cummins' particular scenario you may or may not have noticed that she had a good support strategy i.e. her family. So, a combination of things worked for her, but most of all her own willpower worked the best, along with her strategy in order to prevent the temptation in the first place.

Maintaining a healthy weight

Consider a small example. If you don't take proper care of your car on a regular basis, if you refuse to fuel it whenever the need be or if you turn a blind eye to signals, would your car look good or run properly? No! The same applies for your body; therefore, you must maintain it at all times.

Solution

Start with changing your mindset about dieting. People often confuse dieting as being a tool to lose weight, which is completely false. What is needed is a healthy level of weight to attain, which you have to work and maintain yourself regularly. As you always have to look after your car to ensure a smooth run, you must take care of your body at all times as well.

"Motivation is the art of getting people to do what you want them to do because they want to do it"

- Dwight D Eisenhower

The power of reframing

If something out of your control happens there may still be a reason for it, but you must dig deep to find it. Self-searching for the correct answer is an art that you too can master, look and keep searching until you find the true reason. Your mind however, may play tricks on you from time to time, and therefore won't always let you think how you should be thinking. Changing your mindset to one that knows only the correct answer is the only way to be successful. Your job is to stay on course with your true beliefs and values, and your thought process should remain intact at all times. If for some reason something doesn't go quite to plan, then you must immediately search for a positive outcome which matches your desire(s), and at all times you must stick with your pre-set goals and the task at hand.

According to four psychology professors, (academic board) of The Mind Gym (2005), when you have a stressful situation you can try reframing. Reframing can better prepare you for days when you feel like things aren't quite going your way. Below is one strategy you can use.

Potential thought – I'm trying my best, but I don't seem to be losing any weight.

Reframe – "There's only one strategy to lose weight successfully and it involves the combination of the mind and body. I have all of the answers within this book so I

107

(now/will soon) know what i have to do in order to get what I want".

Potential thought – I'm never going to reach my goal weight.

Reframe – "When I reach each process goal that I have set for myself I am going to appreciate it all the more for all the challenges I've had to overcome to get to that particular point".

Potential thought – I've got such a long way to go it seems an impossible task to do everything I need to do.

Reframe – "Each task that I have set for myself is realistic and achievable, but I know it is a step-by-step process. Every positive thought that I have is one step closer to an action that'll lead me to better health. Losing weight is a positive by-product of eating sensibly and being more active, my life is now how it is meant to be – healthy."

Self-talk

If you continuously find it difficult to change your internal self-talk dialogue then perhaps you need to analyse it and figure out exactly what it is you are saying to yourself.

Sarah Litvinoff (2004) asks you to do the following:
1. List the negative things you habitually say to yourself
2. Play with the voices (say the phrase out loud but in a funny voice, or even play with the volume)
3. Ban the phrases (hush the noise completely).

Recognising what you are saying to yourself allows you to do something about it. After all, if it affects your self-confidence in a negative way why wouldn't you want to change it?

Now is the time to implant good messages:
   1. Choose the best phrase for you and your weight loss success
From all the tasks and all your findings from each chapter choose any positive and uplifting affirmations that give your self-esteem a boost. Combine and involve your new beliefs related to your mind and body i.e. your thoughts, actions and behaviours specific to nutrition and exercise. Try and use future tense as if you already have what you want and do what you set out to do. Soon you will discover more about visualisation, imagery, etc and these will enable you to blend your phrases using the techniques you have found most resourceful.
   2. Repeat the phrases 20 times each morning

A summarised phrase or phrases of the above can be shouted out, repeated silently to yourself or written down, whatever works best for you.

    3.   Say it with conviction

Strength and certainty are key words here, so long as you believe in what you are putting out there.

    4.   Notice the results

It will come with practice but keep a check on your feelings throughout the whole process.

    5.   Take the phrase out with you

This exercise can be practiced anywhere and at anytime.

Sarah Litvinoff sets golden rules for you to abide by:

- Always look for the simplest actions you can take first. So look at each task as you would an exam question, and if you can do it immediately then do so, but if not go back to it later.
- As you attempt each task and/or carry out an action monitor your energy levels related to your confidence.

If you don't expect too much of yourself, and you are realistic about your current abilities you will begin to feel that you can actually do more to be successful and fulfilled, not forgetting happier and more relaxed.

You can gradually increase the amount of affirmations if you choose, but for now try the following:

1. Start with one affirmation that summarises what you want. Repeat this until you feel you are on the correct path.
2. Break your summarised affirmation down into more specific chunks (thoughts/nutrition/physical) and increase the amount you have according to how much detail you want to use.

These can be spread out throughout the day in order to enhance the whole experience, and their timings can relate to when you feel that you will most require them. In other words, use as many as you can and as many times as you can until each specific change is permanent.

Action thoughts

An important aspect of your life is self-realisation, and this can assist you in the following ways:

- Having more control over your thoughts
- Being more responsible for your actions
- Making yourself more accountable, to ensure your future success.

These processes will help you to control the way you live your life from this moment on, and once you establish self-realisation of your thoughts and actions then this can assist you in establishing how successful you are going to be.

💡 Think about a common thought that you have that goes against what you want.
- Write down how this thought made you feel, and how it influenced the way you behaved?
- Write down how this thought limits your actions, and what may be a more helpful way of thinking?

Live and breathe positive psychology
When you master the art of positive thinking it almost guarantees that you have that 'feel-good factor' throughout every moment of your day. Along with healthy food, regular exercise and sufficient rest, these positive thoughts can keep you on the right path towards your weight loss success. Your thoughts lead not only to a feeling, but also to a physiological change in your body. Positive people frequently have a high degree of physical robustness and resilience, says Lynn Williams (2009).

It's so easy however to get caught up with negative thought patterns, especially when you start talking about the weather, and the trouble in the world, etc. Lynn Williams continues to say that there's no denying that you need energy and resilience to do the things you want to do and to maintain a positive outlook on life.

Change the way you think, change the way you are

Remember that eating nutritious foods and exercising on a daily basis should keep any low moments to a bare minimum, but let's address your thoughts. When you feel low you need to think of all the good things that are going on in your life.

💡 Write down all the *good things* that are going on in your life and keep these close to you for anytime that you may feel low.

Pre-plan for those bumps along the way

Being optimistic is just about being positive in the knowledge that you have covered all areas so that nothing stands in your way. We all have days where if we want to eat something high in calories then we can. What we must do, however, is to have in our minds that this does not have to be a 'bad day', because prior to this we would have planned our strategy.

See example below.

Off Course (examples)	Prearranged Strategy (within 12hrs prior)	Prearranged Strategy (within 12hrs after)
Pre-planned – I will decide to have a dessert whilst eating out with friends	I will work out for longer (than normal)	Unplanned – I will do an extra workout – or do a longer workout & I will work harder (than normal)
Pre-planned – I will watch TV for longer than planned tomorrow night	I will go for a longer walk (than normal) at a faster pace prior to the TV fest	Unplanned – I will do an extra walk or do a longer walk & at a faster pace (than normal)

First of all you must ensure that your plan is achievable; therefore, progressive and then you must ensure that you are prepared for any distractions i.e. planning for the what if this or that happens scenario?

Having strategies to use to deal with circumstances that might possibly go wrong with your weight loss plan can be an effective tool for dealing with unexpected problems. For example:
- What if you are running late for work, your alarm didn't go off and you cannot eat your healthy breakfast? What's your plan B?
- What if your personal trainer cancels or your gym class is postponed? What's your plan B?
- What if you don't feel up to exercising on a particular day, you are not sick but your motivation levels are lower than normal? What are you going to do?
- What if you are round a friend's house for a party and they don't have any healthy options for you to eat? Do you know how to say no, or do you have a strategy for times like this?

What you will do in times of feeling:
- Isolated – call a relative on the phone
- Lonely – visit a friend
- Stressed out – go and do something you enjoy doing (hobby, etc.).

If you don't have support, seek out a health care professional who can assist you, contact a local support group, etc.

These strategies can then be fine-tuned and rehearsed mentally. Most people already know what may or may not keep them on track, but be rest assured, you can get back on track with a pre-planned strategy.

10 tips for making new habits and breaking old habits:

1. Visualisation – Success should be visualised, and the trick is to place your-self in the position you want to be in for example, fitting into smaller clothes, enjoying a healthier body, feeling more energetic, or even looking good in the gym or in a similar environment. You should keep the focus to complete all the steps that are necessary to reach the desired stage. You should feel happy, successful and accomplished in your journey of break-ing old habits; feel as if you already have what you want.

2. Inner exploration – Any kind of discomfort should be explored and you should figure out what the reason is that doesn't enable you to make the desired change. You should consider if you feel more comfortable being fat and unhealthy. Maybe your idea of achieving your goal of being thin is frightening? Every moment in the process of breaking old habits, you should think why there is some resistance to this change. In most cases, it is only laziness and lack of self-discipline, but in some cases it may be something serious that happens in the psyche. To get out of this kind of discomfort and resistance you can spend some time in peace, meditation or prayer.

3. Small steps – A single step at a time. Although everything should depend on what your desired state is i.e. if your goal is to lose 10st, then the pro-cess should always start with small steps. The first thing is to get assistance and then for you to sign a contract of accountability ensuring you under-stand about your tasks (short and long-term). Then comes taking small steps, one day at a time doing. Or whatever it takes in order to achieve permanent weight loss success. At this point in time, you should not think about the past or what didn't work for you before. The thing to think of is short-term future goals, and by one step at a time you will be able to break old habits.

4. Trying to make changes that are symbolic. Even simple things like:
   - Getting a makeover
   - Buying better fitting clothes
   - Sitting in a healthier restaurant while dining
   - Walking somewhere to have lunch rather than ordering fast food or going to a drive thru
   - Concentrating on your posture, walk tall and proud through healthy living
   - Changing the arrangement of your daily routine can also help.

All these little things could symbolise the much bigger change in your life that you are looking for.

112

5.   Your progress should be celebrated – There should be celebration with some of the steps, be it losing your 1st pound of body fat or anything similar. It is all about enjoying the small steps you are taking during your attempt to make new habits, and so you should be rewarded; therefore, celebrate each milestone you set for yourself.

6.   Awareness of your actions – It has to be ensured that the actions you take and your new behaviour correspond with your goals when you are trying to get out of your old habits. For example, if you want to lose weight, you have to think twice before you finish the whole of a banana split or pack of crisps or biscuits. Or, if you want a new body, you should invest in managing your time better. Changing your exercise and nutrition habits rather than being a couch potato and watching TV every spare moment you get. Your energy should be channelled and very focused if you want to make new long-lasting habits. It's all about choice.

7.   The end result should be on focus – Although it depends on personality, it may become too overwhelming for you. In this case it may help if you can remember why you are breaking old habits i.e. of being a specific weight category. You should think about your goal on a daily basis if you have to make new habits.

8.   Your thoughts should be monitored – If you have the mentality of 'all or nothing', you have to get out of that way of thinking. For example, you should make sure you do not think that eating a couple of cookies could create problems if you are maintaining a routine to lose weight. Experience and logic should be used in the long run to break your old habits, make new ones, and to maintain the new ones. If you do have a high calorie treat then just ensure that you make up for it when you are exercising, but don't punish yourself mentally.

9.   Joining a formal support system – Belonging to a formal system like this helps you to follow a healthier and more positive routine. For example, when it comes to doing more exercise, you can go and buy a bunch of exercise packages like yoga, spinning, body pump or even some personal training sessions to help you during the initial phase. The idea is also to make friends and build a new network of like-minded positive people. As previously mentioned it is very important and advisable to make connections with a fitness specialist, someone who can also advise you on nutrition, etc. related to your goals and aspirations.

10. Your mind, body and soul should be nurtured – This is extremely important and should be taken care of instantly. You should also sleep enough if you are trying to make your new habits take place. Not only should you eat nutritious food and spend quality time looking after yourself, but you should also enjoy life and be happy.

113

"Challenge your lifestyle, and make yourself accountable for the rest of your days."

- Wellness FitCoach

What exactly is your plan?
Make yourself aware that this is a plan that needs 110% of your energy; it's a daily thing, every second, and every minute you must think about your future health.

♥Task 27
Go and get your notebook and pen!
Write down at least 10 things that you are prepared to do to succeed:

1. ....
2. ....
3. ....
4. ....
5. ....
6. ....
7. ....
8. ....
9. ....
10. ....

How to get out of your comfort zone

Change the goal posts
Why is changing eating habits or sticking to an exercise routine so difficult? While external and genetic factors play a role, you are ultimately in charge of your daily decisions about what to eat and how much to do physically. So why do you find yourself falling back into old eating habits? And why is changing your eating habits so difficult?

♥Task 28
List the times when you wanted to do something, but refrained from doing it for some reason or another:

1. ....
2. ....
3. ....
4. ....
5. ....

Average person example:
I was thinking about joining a gym, but I never went because I didn't want to be seen by anyone, I also didn't want to feel uneasy around all those fit-looking people.

Now describe times when you stepped out of your comfort zone i.e. you wanted to do something so badly, it took you some time to work yourself up to it but you just went for it:

1. ....
2. ....
3. ....
4. ....
5. ....

Average person comes good example:
I was given a free 'trial' membership to my local gym and I'm so glad I went as I've had some great results. I was amazed at how many other people are in there just like me. I replaced sitting in front of the TV watching chat shows with getting a step closer to achieving my dreams, all from changing an unnecessary habit and stepping out of my comfort zone.

Understanding what affects your self-confidence

*"I figured that if I said it enough, I would convince the world that
I really was the greatest."*

- Mohammad Ali

Once you begin to raise your emotional intelligence, it can be very rewarding for you and likewise, it will substantially increase your confidence. Your confidence needs to support you throughout the whole weight loss process; therefore, you must constantly manage it for full effectiveness.

♥Task 29
Low confidence situations
List all the situations or circumstances that sometimes cause your confidence to diminish:

1. ....
2. ....
3. ....
4. ....
5. ....

Take these and turn them into positives by listing how you can regain confidence.

High confidence situations
List all the situations regarding weight loss that you feel completely confident:

1. ....
2. ....

115

3. ....

4. ....

5. ....

Now recreate the mental state associated with permanent weight loss success!

Visualisation

Make your dream a visual reality

Visualisation not only relaxes you but it is also a good way of coping with any stress you may have. Try not to be too judgmental though, by over analyzing your vision, as it may restrict what you are trying to achieve. But you can most certainly manipulate your brain via visualisation by focusing your mind on a pleasant vision that is enthusiastic and supportive of your goal.

These types of visions will completely relax your body, make you feel physically lighter and fill you full of energy. Scientific research suggests that effective visualisation increases your chances of achieving your goals, and by many it is deemed as one of the strongest mental 'tools' at your disposal. Through association your mind converts images to whatever specific meaning they have to you, and certain images can therefore trigger emotional and/or physical responses due to them feeling real to you. Even though it is called visualisation the more senses you use the more real your vision will be i.e. you can also include sound, touch, taste and even smell.

For example, imagine yourself looking and feeling fantastic, you have the body to die for and everyone around you are admiring how you look. You hear people talking about you, you can feel the slender tone of your body, and you smell like a million dollar bottle of perfume/aftershave.

You can also relate visualisation to nutrition if you want to i.e. imagine eating something you know is good for you (a fruit or veg that you normally find difficult to eat). For example, fruits that taste so fresh due to them just being picked from the tree, they have a smooth texture yet the sound of you biting into it is distinct, and the smell is so fruity it makes your mouth water for more.

The same goes for exercise and anything else that you deem to be a barrier for you. If you want to develop the habit of going to the gym, you can build positive images about how great you feel as you get ready, as you workout and as you finish the session. Positive images can be reinforced with detailed messages around your specific behaviours and it's up to you how you want to adopt these.
Of course the feeling after exercise is like no other, so this needs to be enhanced too.

You can also add contrast to your images, depth and even movement too. If your vision has emotion it should only be positive, and it should always make you happy.

116

As previously mentioned, the feeling you require is one of satisfaction, a feeling that you already possess what you desire. Whilst visualising consider your breathing too, but above all ensure you keep practicing as this makes for perfection, so be extremely patient with this particular strategy.

Basics of Visualisation

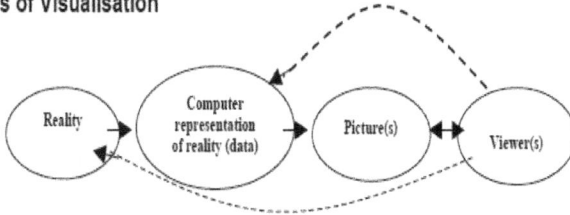

It is critical that when you start the Lifestyle Challenge and throughout the 21 days (non-stop) thereafter, you establish a new pattern in your brain by focusing on and repeating the following thought processes. Remember that your mind has accepted how you are today because of your vision. Your personal picture never had the opportunity to change until now.

Visualisation (Mental imagery)
Program the non-conscious part of your mind and see yourself in your minds eye – not as you are now but how you would ideally like to be. If you do this on a daily basis and for a minimum of 21 days (non-stop), this will become an automatic process.

To make it easier, picture it as putting new grooves on a record by replacing the old (negative) grooves with a view that, in time, the old negative thoughts will be taken over by brand new positive ones. For ease, find pictures from magazines or books of what you would like to look like and place them somewhere you can see them on a daily basis. If you have a computer, shrink or enlarge them and print them off and carry them everywhere with you. Place them wherever you can see them but remember, do not move on until you have done this. You will be well on your way to success once you have prepared your mind because your body will want to follow.

♥Task 30
Visualisation
Hold and concentrate on a picture in your mind of how you would like something to be. To visualise losing weight, you need to hold a picture in your mind of your ideal body, whether it is by using an old photograph or a magazine picture, to help you visualise. The clearer your picture is, the more successful you will be and only then can you spend some time each day thinking of yourself as already having and owning what your image is portraying – this new, improved you.

Over time, this will bring you closer to your weight loss goals by working on your subconscious mind to achieve the desired results. Suddenly fast food, sweets, cans of Coke and all those desserts will seem less tempting and long walks will seem more fun, but only because of what is in line with the 'set point' you are visualising.

117

"Action is the real measure of intelligence."

- Napoleon Hill

Use your imagination

☀ Imagine clearly the following:
- Your ideal bodyweight (as if you already have it)
- Your ideal body image (as above).

Maintenance – throughout each and every day (for 21 days) maintain these images in your mind.

Result – your subconscious mind will bring forth the actions necessary to make it into your reality.

Transformation – your imagination can transform your life and your body without you having to consciously make the tough decisions necessary to do so.

Choice – your imagination and new subconscious choices can assist you in the following ways:
- Ensures you make better food choices
- Ensures you move your body more often.

Using your imagination properly can make you do all this without you having to think and plan too much, after 21 days it will become automatic.

Have a go!

Relaxation phase
Close your eyes, take a deep relaxing breath in and out.

Picture perfect phase
Picture or imagine the ideal version of you, and once you see that image, begin to visualise every aspect of it. Get a clear-cut image of your entire body from your feet all the way up to the smile on your face. Even notice what clothes you're wearing and the background of where you see yourself.

Movement phase
The final step is to put some movement into your image, just like you're the star in your own short film clip. Visualise this every single day as often as possible and begin to notice the small changes you accomplished in the previous week.

Recording phase
Write down all the small changes that you have noticed and see how you're now beginning to become mentally prepared for permanent weight loss success!

If you're having a difficult time imagining or envisioning yourself at your ideal bodyweight, a qualified Clinical Hypnotherapist can help. Best of luck on your life-transforming endeavour!

Control

♥Task 31
<u>Situations where you have no control</u>
List all the situations regarding weight loss that you feel completely out of control:

1. ....
2. ....
3. ....
4. ....
5. ....

Take these and turn them into positives by listing how you can regain control.

<u>Situations where you have control</u>
List all the situations regarding weight loss that you feel completely in control:

1. ....
2. ....
3. ....
4. ....
5. ....

Avoid getting overhelmed

When you think about what you have to do to get what you want, instead of panicking just relax and practice self-reflection and try and remind yourself that you are now in a better place. You should now be able to stop and think about yourself and observe and evaluate whether your thoughts are rational and helpful. You should now be in possession of the following:

- Increased confidence
- Controlled happiness
- Increased awareness about spirit and meaning (law of attraction, gratitude, etc)
- More in tune with your mind (thoughts, behaviours and actions)
- Increased knowledge about how to achieve set goals
- You should be more competent than when you first started.

You should now be able to identify the thoughts that you experience and these should be both:
- Rational and logical.

You should also be able to:

- Put each situation into perspective.

For example, people who have lost weight before or people who do not have an issue with gaining weight, ask yourself 'is this the way they would think, or how might they approach my situation?'

You should also be able to:
- Identify if your thoughts are helpful to you in order to accomplish each task.

Ensure that you have prioritised everything in a logical manner i.e. your planning and structured program (mind, nutrition and exercise-wise) has been thought through enough right down to the finer details. Your thoughts should be constructive, self-supportive and ones that are helpful. They also need to be reinforced frequently so as to build new habits as and when required.

Below is an example of a simple version of a daily plan.

Tomorrow I plan to do the following:

8am – wake up and begin my self-talk (continue it approx. every hour)
- *Prepare breakfast & lunch the night before*, to save you time in the morning
- Get up a little bit earlier than normal and *put on PT kit that is beside my bed*
- Complete 15 minutes of exercise, good warm up but high intensity
- Get showered
- Have breakfast *prepared the night before*
- Go to work
- Have lunch *prepared the night before*
- Return home
- Complete 15 minutes of exercise
- Have dinner *prepared the night before*
- Plan meals, etc. for the next day
- Relax.

9pm – go to bed, and complete my final self-talk for the day (adjust dialogue if required)

Repeat each day, each week for 21 days non-stop.*

As you can imagine you can go into even more detail by planning the ingredients of your meals, your exercise sessions and also add in your self-talk dialogue (explained later). For ease, we kept it simple.

*If you stop, just carry that day over – simple.

IMPORTANT

Nine times out of ten you may find that your TV, play station or checking social media/lounging around time will have to be reduced significantly in order to get what you want. If this is the case then you have to decide what is important to you. According to Mihaly Csikszentmihaly (1997), watching TV, is probably the most novel form of activity in human experience, yet there is no development of the 'self'. He goes on to mention that according to Greek philosophers it is during leisure that we become truly human by devoting time to self-development.

If your work hours are so long, then you may have to mention your health worries to your boss, stating that you need to have a longer lunch break or finish work early. Say or do anything in order to exercise more as this is about you, your health, reducing stress and living longer. Most issues today are related to poor time management and poor lifestyle habits that need to be broken. Remember, where there's a will there's always a way.

Write down your day as it should be, to include:
1. Your own self-talk dialogue (more examples given later)
2. Planning the ingredients of your meals
3. Your exercise sessions.

Before you commence your 21-day plan ensure you have the following in check:
1. Your beliefs and values
2. Your thoughts and expectations
3. Your emotions, behaviours and actions.

To support the above, we have written the above in lay terms related to what you should have covered within this book:
*   All tasks completed
*   Your outcome goal highlighted (target weight/realistic timescale, etc.)
*   Your daily process goals (realistic and achievable milestones of progress)
*   Your daily self-talk dialogue (positive words that will motivate you to take action)
*   Your action plan (strategies for all eventualities that could go wrong)
*   Your positive resources (thoughts/food/exercise – choices to replace not-so-good habits)
*   Your support team fully briefed and informed of your plan (on standby with punishments)
*   Your start date in order to complete 21 days non-stop (realistic and achievable).

♥Task 32
Now that you've read this much of the book ensure you do the following:
1. Answer: What makes you think you are more motivated today than ever before?

121

2. Choose a realistic date and specific time of day when you will start your exercise plan and tell everyone you know about it too
3. Restock your kitchen with nutritious food and drink
4. Invest in your health and select the vitamins and minerals that you need
5. Put together a list of food and juice menus for the forthcoming week
6. Purchase exercise clothes from training shoes to an all-weather tracksuit
7. Select an exercise plan
8. Make everyday an awareness day by updating your diary
9. Be more positive about your time management
10. Attract positivity and happiness on all levels
11. Maintain your motivation, especially when the going gets tough
12. Carry inspirational photos/memoirs/quotes, etc. everywhere you go
13. Reassess the things you *feel* you cannot change
14. Always be on the lookout for alternatives that taste the same
15. Find the time and money to go organic/low GI as quick as you can.

"Create a new mental state that you can now associate with permanent weight loss success!"

- Wellness FitCoach

Wellness FitCoach rule

Alter a negative thought before you action or behave in a manner that is not congruent with your plan. Override something about your life that is negative or not in line with your values in order for change to take place. For example, the way you look at food and think about exercise.

Feel-good factor
The advantage of having a pen and paper on hand is that when you feel good, whether it is because of what you are wearing or what physical activity you have just done, is so that you can write down how you felt or 'capture it in a bottle' as they say. Everything you sense can then be recreated as your optimal mindset for the future.

Be responsible for your own happiness.

What we must do is achieve happiness first, and this will increase your chance of being successful in the future.
Rules:
1. Forget about the past, forget about tomorrow and just focus on what you are going to do today!
2. You must be realistic about temptations, because somewhere along the way you will eventually cheat on your plan. Once you accept this, you can be at peace when it eventually happens, and you may even have a strategy that will help you prepare for it too.

3. Irrespective of whether your strategy to overcome temptation works or not, the best way to prepare is by *accepting* the fact that it's happened, *forgiving yourself* for the moment, and then *maintaining control* over the situation in order to get back on track.

"The happiest people in the world are those who feel absolutely terrific about themselves, and this is the natural outgrowth of accepting total responsibility for every part of their life."

- Brian Tracy

Summary

In this book we have been mainly focusing on weight loss itself, which is very important but what we tend to forget is that it is overall health that we should be focusing on. Even though contributing factors to death are all interlinked in some way, we should still look at the real causes of heart disease:
- Eating Trans fats (artificially hydrogenated oils)
- Cooking with heavily refined vegetable oils, such as soy, cottonseed, corn oil, etc. They are inflammatory inside the body and typically throw the omega-6/omega-3 balance out of whack
- Eating too much refined sugar in the diet, including high fructose corn syrup
- Eating too much refined carbohydrates, such as white bread and low fiber cereals
- Smoking
- Leading a stressful lifestyle
- A lack of exercise
- Other lifestyle factors.

Apart from smoking, heart disease and being overweight have the same contributing factors, so if this means making small improvements to your meals and your habits until they feel natural and a part of your new mode of thinking, then you'll surely reap the benefits forever. When the time comes and your stomach is saying I need food, you have to give it something and it will be down to you what you give it.

The secret to success for maintaining an optimum weight is eating a little now when you first feel hungry rather than a lot more later when you're truly starving.

Snacking
Is the best way to maintain your blood sugar and weight. Some people think snacking is cheating or ruining your appetite, but all you are doing is eating in a measured way all the time. Healthy snacking keeps you from bingeing on a huge dinner after starving yourself all day.

Why do you think it is that you see the skinny girl in the corner nearly always eating? The choices you make, as important as they are, will reflect on how you feel,

123

how you function and if you know in your heart of hearts that those choices were better than before, then and only then are you on your way to winning.

Enjoy Moving:
- Instead of heading to the fridge, put on one of your favorite songs, grab your training shoes, and do a few sets of all over body exercises.
- Need a change of scenery? Embrace yard work. Mowing the lawn with a push mower and digging in the garden will all get your muscles working. Do anything you can.
- Maintaining a regular yoga practice can enhance your weight-loss regimen, primarily by toning muscles and reducing stress. If this is your new choice of activity, aim to practice for at least one hour, two times a week and varying the type of yoga you do, from gentle to more intense styles.
- At this stage you shouldn't be thinking of any excuses, you should be on the road to being positive with the smart strategies that you have just re-vealed, strategies that you can ultimately start to adopt now.
- You should be thinking about boosting the intensity of your daily life with quality foods and safe exercises, completed with a good attitude and a real-istic frame of mind.
- You should try and use your common sense at all times throughout the program.
-

For example, walking up hills is better than on flat ground and swinging your arms across your chest will be better than not. Swimming is free and great on the joints. Why not do something fun while getting in great shape at the same time? Maybe you could start hiking mountains or take up cross country skiing, snowshoeing or downhill skiing. The activity you choose is more than just fun and when the weather warms up, perhaps you could try out water sports like kayaking or canoeing or take up mountain biking.

Remember: Strength training has greater implications for decreasing body fat and sustaining fat free mass. Adding exercise programs to dietary restriction can pro-mote more favorable changes in body composition than diet or physical activity on its own.

Road to Success:
- Eat healthily regularly
- Cut out the JUNK carbohydrates and fats
- Eat good old-fashioned home cooking and avoid takeaway or ready meals that began in a science lab
- Baking, boiling, steaming and stir-frying are examples of heart-healthy cooking
- Stop eating before you become stuffed full and uncomfortable
- Never go hungry, you'll find yourself nibbling on everything that comes your way, and don't skip meals

124

- Eat a piece of fruit on the way to the restaurant to put that appetite under control.

Remember: That it's just the little things. As an example, the average American is gaining a pound a year and did you know that is the result of eating just 10 extra calories a day?
So, instead of depriving yourself of all your favorites, continue to enjoy them every once in while. It's the little things that will make a difference. If you must have butter, have it on one slice not two. If you must have your caffeine, get used to black coffee. Stop at the 10th chip not the whole bag, at least it will be justified.

Calories in, calories out
To lose weight, you have to cut down on the number of calories you consume and start burning more calories each day. Calories are the amount of energy in the food you eat and some foods have more calories than others. But, foods high in fat and sugar are also typically high in calories. If you eat more calories than your body uses, the extra calories will be stored as excess body fat. Making the transition from a bad-fat diet to a good-fat diet is more easy than you would think. All you have to do is minimise your consumption of meat, full-fat dairy products, fast food, and products made with partially hydrogenated oils, vegetable shortening, and common vegetable oils.

Keep it realistic and achievable at this stage so that it doesn't become a chore but ultimately it becomes a natural part of your day. This first 21 days are the most important.

All of the Lifestyle Challenges should be incorporated into your new daily routine to include:
1. Reasons why you want to lose weight
2. Positive thinking
3. Visualisation
4. Goal setting
5. New food choices.

Your present motivation level will dictate when to start your Lifestyle Challenges and incorporate them into your daily routine. It's pretty much down to you but the timing has to be right, if not perfect.

Michael Van Straten, author of Super Energy Detox explains that "you should just focus on putting one foot in front of the other and you'll be surprised at how quickly you become absorbed in what you're doing, and that will be the beginning of the regeneration of your energy." If you think it will help, re-read the book but you must adopt *ALL* of the strategies. If you remember nothing else, remember this, something that I will never forget my grandfather saying to me, "No one person who has already achieved what they want in this life are any kind of supermen or superwomen. They are not special in any way, shape or form. Of course they had

125

motivation and the willpower to carry on, but we are all born with the same make-up."

"The saddest summary of a life contains three descriptions: could have, might have, and should have."

- Louis E. Boone

<u>Understanding everything that this book has tried to portray</u>
Understand more about:
- What causes your self-confidence to wane
- Visualisation techniques
- Positive self-talk.

<u>Courage</u>
The things that you *think* you can't do, pluck up the courage to have a go at them anyway and see how it feels. I speak from experience when I say "you won't be disappointed".

Task checklist

Part 5: Combining it all
☐ ♥ Task 27
Write down at least 10 things that you are prepared to do to succeed.
☐ ♥ Task 28
List the times when you wanted to do something, but refrained from doing them for some reason or another.
☐ ♥ Task 29
Low and high confidence situations.
☐ ♥ Task 30
Visualisation.
☐ ♥ Task 31
Control situations.
☐ ♥ Task 32
Now that you've read this much of the book ensure you do the following…

Part 6: EXTRA TOOLS

"Courage and perseverance have a magical talisman, before which difficulties disappear and obstacles vanish into air."

- John Quincy Adams

In the following chapter there are some useful tools and information you may find helpful. It is not essential to complete all of these, but by implementing some or all of them might aid you on your weight loss journey.

Planning your own strategy

In addition to your daily plan, the following is an example of how you might add in other useful tools found in this book to help you during your day.

Understanding what affects your self-confidence
Firstly you must stabilise your confidence by creating awareness.

High confidence situations	Low confidence situations
List all the situations with weight loss in which you feel completely confident	List all the situations or circumstances that sometimes cause your confidence to diminish.
1.	1.
2.	2.
etc.	etc.

"Confidence is contagious. So is a lack of confidence."

-Vince Lombardi

Visualisation
Do the following in order to bridge the gap between your ability and your confidence.

The spotlight – Imagine a huge spotlight beaming down on the floor in front of you.
Your ideal self – If you have been your ideal weight before, go back to that time and place; however, if not…think about the weight that you would like to be, with a body that you would be more than happy with. Wearing the clothes that you would like to wear now, doing the things that you would like to do now. Think about how positive and confident you were/would be, everything you did/do was/is effortless.
From the outside looking in – Imagine now that you are looking at yourself from the outside and see yourself actually inside the circle of the spotlight. Imagine exactly

127

what the 'you' inside the circle is seeing, hearing, feeling and smelling. Notice the taste of weight loss success in your mouth.

The spotlight is now on you – Now step into the spotlight and become fully associated so that you are experiencing events through your own eyes and in real time. Again, notice what you are seeing, hearing, feeling, smelling and tasting.

Imagery and self-hypnosis
A good way to develop this particular skill is to recreate the image of a celebrity you like, someone that inspires you and you would like to be like and fully imagine yourself as that person. So long as they are a positive role model i.e. they eat healthily and exercise, etc.

The more senses you involve, the better the success rate i.e. adding sounds, smells and feelings too.

Calm before the storm
In order to assist you to feeling 'up for it' let your imagination go wild by practicing the following *2-3 minutes per day*:
1. Sit in a comfy chair
2. Relax
3. Close your eyes
4. Breathe slowly and deeply
5. As you exhale allow the tension and stress to leave your muscles.

Distance your mind from the here and now and place yourself in a place that you associate with relaxation and inner calm. The power of doing this is incredible, especially prior to starting your day or when you get home from work. But more importantly it will give you a boost prior to eating healthily and doing some form of physical activity. This is also an incredible way to block out any nagging doubts that may have crept into your mind; therefore, re-focus on your task of losing weight.

Emotionally-focussed goal setting
The goal setting process works best when:
• There is some form of flexibility
• You take ownership of each goal, each and every day.

Goal setting has been found to be an effective intervention strategy designed to control unhelpful emotions. You will now have become more aware of your emotions, and it is at this point you need to set emotionally focused goals. When your emotions start to become unhelpful to you, using such effective strategies will assist you to control and change these emotions.

Your desire to change is crucial

By the end of January the mass population who decided to set goals of losing weight have failed. Such goals code-named 'New Years resolutions' become typical examples of how not to set goals. It makes you wonder if the real reason behind such goals are because such like-minded individuals know that they are going to overindulge and just need a reason to do that. 'I'm eating and drinking to excess because I am going to lose it next year' – consequently setting themselves up for more weight gain, more heartache and more stress!

Anyone can achieve significant improvements in their lives by means of effective goal setting, and if you have the following you will stand more chance of success:
- Mental strength
- A clear vision of exactly what you want to achieve
- A plan of how to get there.

Goal setting is a powerful technique that works if you have the following:
- A direction for your efforts
- Focus
- Persistence
- Confidence.

Your confidence will support you throughout the whole weight loss process, but it needs to be constantly managed.

Principles of setting goals and how to apply them effectively

In order to attain the confidence required to be successful you need to inspire yourself and give yourself a target to aim for. The goals you set for yourself must be specific, measurable, achievable, recorded, time framed, evaluated and reversible:

- *Specific* – What exactly do you want to achieve?
- *Measurable* – Can you quantify it? Example, to lose 100lb
- *Achievable* – Is it realistically achievable and accepted as worthwhile for you?
- *Recorded* – As you write down your goals form a contract with yourself
- *Time framed* – Have you set yourself a specific time limit? Example, 6 months/1 year
- *Evaluated* – Are you monitoring your progress regularly?
- *Reversible* – Are you able and pre-prepared to adjust/reset your goals in the event of injury or negative moments?

Thought Process
- Establish your own vision of what you want to achieve.

Planning Process
- Plan how you are going to achieve this goal with realistic day-to-day tasks.
So that you don't get overwhelmed, you must keep it simple by taking small steps in order to achieve your dream goal.

129

For example:

Choose 1 Dream Goal (long-term) – this year I want to lose 100lb – get excited that this can and will happen, but don't get too stressed by focussing on it too much.

Choose 2-3 Intermediate Goals – within 6 months I want to lose 50lb, fit into clothes 3 sizes smaller and be able to take part in a 5km fun run for charity – these goals are more flexible and within your control but should remain meaningful and realistic.

Choose 2 Short-term Goals – to eat healthy and do some form of physical activity each and every day (in order to lose 2.2lb or 1kg each week).

As you can see the short-term goals are your highest priority and your most important actions that are required to achieve success. They provide you with focus on a day-to-day basis, and if you can get this part right you will naturally progress towards your intermediate goals; therefore, be well on your way to permanent weight loss success.

Small Steps for Bigger results
So, what we need to do now is make a decision on the following…

What do you need to do each and every day in order to succeed?
This ultimately relates to what habits you are willing to change and what choices you are prepared to make. But whatever you decide, you will be a small step closer towards your next intermediate goal, and ultimately towards your dream goal.

Intrinsic motivation
Our aim is for you to be in harmony with your sense of self, and your new goals and habits to be almost entirely self-determined. This motivation comes from within, it is fully self-determined and characterised by interest in and enjoyment from participation in the task you have set for yourself:
- To know
- To accomplish
- To experience stimulation.

Intrinsic motivation is considered to be the healthiest type of motivation.

Reward yourself for your short-term successes
The key aspect of rewards is to reinforce your sense of competence and self-worth; the reward you choose should be informational in nature rather than controlling in order to avoid undermining your intrinsic motivation. Therefore, avoid rewards that have too much monetary value. For example, if you joined a weight loss group or have your own personal trainer/life coach they can present you (in front of all other participants) with a token reward i.e. most successful weight loss (this week) award or similar. Also, if you don't have any outside assistance then you could buy yourself a new outfit for exercise or for a special event, etc.

130

Your formula for improved motivation

To determine the motivational qualities of an individual piece of music you need to recognise how your emotions change when you hear certain types of music. The music should influence you, and your mood state should be one of happiness, which in turn can assist in enhancing your activity levels. The same goes for video footage. Will watching a YouTube clip of someone who has lost large amounts of weight give you motivation? Or similarly watching someone who has recovered from heart disease by losing weight or would you watch something completely different? Your chosen footage could be accompanied by your choice of music rather than the music being a separate motivating factor, or you could use both.

Develop Your Confidence

Commit to your own personal vision: For example, I want to lose 2.2lbs or 1kg per week. You must believe that this goal is achievable (which it is) and worth striving for (because these small steps will get you to your dream goal, of course it is). If you have a personal trainer then you must agree this goal with them or make yourself accountable and make an agreement with yourself.

IMPORTANT

Remember that these are small... but realistic steps...closer to your dream goal...also that goals can be adjusted, as long as the reason is to optimise their potential effect on your life.

"It's what you learn after you know it all that counts."

- John Wooden

Don't forget

Consider potential barriers to your goals and plan around them first. Also, ensure you have your pre-planned strategy ready and in your head for when you have bad days, or for when you are sick or injured, etc.

Positive self-talk

This can reinforce your self-esteem and positively alter your belief system. Giving yourself confidence by way of positive self-talk confirms in your own mind that you already possess the building blocks of success to lose weight permanently. Believing in your own ability through your positive attitude and self-belief will ensure you of success, but the statements you use are very important.

Changing Your Dialogue

The fact is you possess an untapped energy source that can be drawn upon to bring about superior results. It's all about the following:
- Changing your attitude
- Having a 'can do' mindset
- Engaging in systematic behaviours.

131

In order to record your emotions you must develop a self-talk diary to run alongside your food and exercise diary. This will assist you in changing your unhelpful emotions into helpful ones. The statements you write will be spoken by you on a daily basis; therefore, they should:

1. Be extremely vivid
2. Roll off your tongue
3. Be 100% believable to you.

"Most importantly it's about the motivation you find from within, and the sense of accomplishment you feel after conquering your goal."

- Kristen Mercier

Time management

For most humans we have this thing about having no time. If time is such a constraint on people's lives why don't we just slow down? My advice to you is to try and be 'in the moment' whenever you can, and this way you can at least cherish everything around you, everything that is being shown to you. So I have devised a strategy for you in order to get you to where you want to get to by using your own thoughts.

At certain times throughout the day, preferably during the times listed overleaf (or alternative times if you work nights), you need to ensure that you are in a place in your head, whereby you can stop time, stop thinking, and shut off all other thoughts from your mind. Whether you stop what you are doing, go to the bathroom or hide in a cupboard. Do whatever you have to do to stop time and reflect on the following headings (or similar headings of your own).

Overleaf I have given you some examples using the times on a clock, and these can be practiced at anytime throughout your day. The words that you use should ideally be your own reflections in order for you to truly connect with them. In the beginning you can start by using the words in the examples, reflecting on one word per day and continue to reflect on that word whenever you remember. In time the idea is for you to connect with a number of words that have personal meaning to you, ones that truly resonate with you and get you the desired results.

Control your thoughts
The overall aim of this self-talk practice is to assist you in creating a natural flow of positive self-talk between your initial thought processes and a positive action outcome. The end product being unconscious continuity of your core values, for the rest of your life.

Mastery of 'self-discipline' (using self-talk)

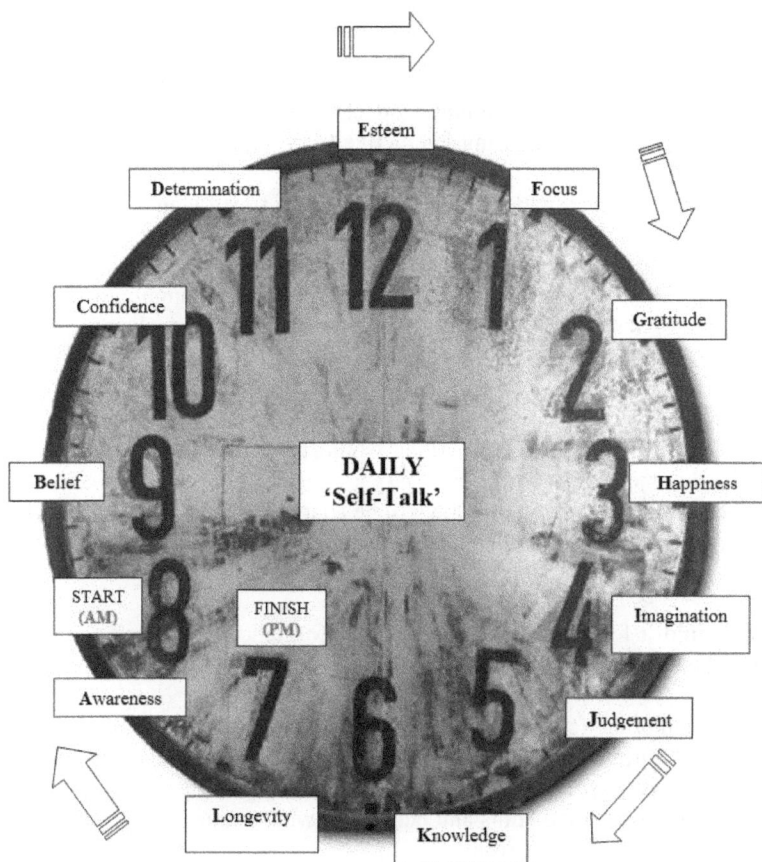

As you can see, by way of <u>an example</u> I have used the alphabet and chosen specific words starting from 8am for each hour until 7pm.

Most of us have that voice in our head that guides us, sometimes with good thoughts, some not so good. It is now time to take control of those thoughts in order to get what you want and use it to your advantage. If used properly and effectively, positive self-talk can help alter your mental state and your receptiveness to the idea of a weight loss programme that will lead you toward long-term, healthy, balanced weight loss.

We propose that for ½ a 24 hour period you do this particular exercise. Despite what time you awake, each hour after you awake you can start your day with our examples or your own and then move to self-talk number 2 etc. Likewise, if you go to bed late you will still finish on self-talk number 12, which in my example is longevity; however, if you wish you could work your way around the clock until you actually go to sleep. My advice would be to choose which words really resonate with you and give you motivation, then insert those in again after number 12.

Conscious of the crucial importance of time? WellnessFitCoach has designed and created a new interactive communication channel, DST technology (Daily Self-Time) which sets up the following interactive loop: Each morning you will receive advice via email and personal support from Wayne Lambert, and every hour after that you will receive a reminder of recommendations specific only to you.

Once you register with www.wellnessfitcoach.com and provide proof of purchase of this book you will then have access to this interactive communication channel. This is a major innovation that only the www.wellnessfitcoach.com site and its Wellness FitCoaches are capable of offering.

This is how it works:
- Your own personal instructions would have taken into account your last daily report
- The information you provide will be adapted to meet your personal needs
- You will get up-to-date and relevant information based on your initial feedback.

So what would it feel like if every piece of information you receive is specific to you only? Just think how much motivation and confidence this will give you.

Being informed of the following information on a daily basis:
- Your current and predicted weight and measurements, keeping you on track every second of the day
- Your current food faults and choices of what you can replace them with for fantastic and speedy results
- Your current motivation levels and how you can keep avoiding any future frustrations
- Your current physical activity levels and how you can progress quicker towards your goals based on your interests and capability.

Positive self-talk
Is not about accomplishing things without having to do anything at all, but rather about motivating yourself to accomplish them. (E.R. Brooks, 2010).

Recognition and control
When you recognise the beginning of a negative emotion you need to have a sentence on hand that you can say to yourself i.e. words in a future tense without any negativity. Some examples you can use are as follows:
- 'Step-by-step I will reach my ideal weight'
- 'Nothing will get in my way of losing weight'
- I can, I will, etc.

Use these or your own, but be sure to write them down yourself and repeat them to yourself every day i.e. when you awake in the morning and before you go to sleep at night. These statements through repetition will become embedded into your mind, and will influence your actions on a daily basis especially during your low-confident moments. You will find that raising your emotional intelligence will be very rewarding and will likewise increase your confidence substantially.

In the following examples, it is planned that you achieve this practice between the hours of 8am-7pm; therefore, upon waking and before you go to sleep. The practice should quite simply be thoughts and self-talk related to your core values and what you want from your life from this moment on. For example, *how you want to feel, etc. rather than just to lose weight.*

You can adjust the timings to suit your routine (for example, if you work nights) but you must adhere to the following actions at specific times throughout your day, and repeat for 21 days.

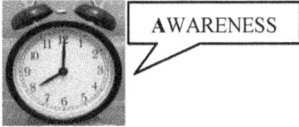
AWARENESS

Good planning and self-control is related to a greater awareness of the vulnerability to health risks and more sensible decisions about diet and exercise. (D.L. Waller, 2011).

Self-talk task
You open your eyes from sleeping at 8am, it's a new day and from this very moment on your thoughts are going to dictate how your day will go. Awareness related to weight loss. Write down at least 10 things related to awareness that will assist you with this practice:

1. ....
2. ....
3. ....
4. ....
5. ....
6. ....
7. ....
8. ....
9. ....
10. ....

Example
I am aware that I have been given a new day to live for, aware of my good health, clean running water, fresh bed clothes, etc. I am aware that however bad I think that

135

something is for me I know that it can still be a lot worse than it is i.e. there is always somebody somewhere worse off than me.

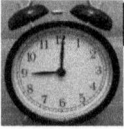

BELIEF

The importance of beliefs in determining health behaviour has been previously incorporated into specific models of health behaviour. These models recognise the importance of a number of personal, environmental and psychosocial factors in determining food choices related to weight loss. (T.P. Starks, 2006).

Self-talk task
It's 9am. Belief related to weight loss. Write down at least 10 things related to belief that will assist you with this practice:
1. ....
2. ....
3. ....
4. ....
5. ....
6. ....
7. ....
8. ....
9. ....
10. ....

Example
I am en route to work and alongside thinking about what I need to do today. I need to collect my thoughts and believe that today will be a good day, even better than yesterday. Believing that I will make good decisions both nutritionally and physically, and that any negative thoughts that come into my head will be turned around into positive, believable thoughts with actions to show for them. I believe that my goals are achievable and worth striving for and these small steps will get me to my dream goal. I don't have a personal trainer yet but when I do I will agree this goal with them, so for now I will make myself accountable and make an agreement with myself.

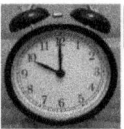

CONFIDENCE

It's 10am. Weight loss is not about fate or luck, it's about adopting a can-do attitude, knowing that you are the person responsible for determining how confident you feel. It is from within your subconscious that most of your motivation will derive. In terms of specific self-confidence interventions, it appears that *motivational self-talk* has a more positive effect on self-confidence than instructional self-talk. (J. Hellenic, 2006).

Self-talk task
Write down at least 10 motivational things related to confidence that will assist you with this practice:
1. ....
2. ....
3. ....
4. ....
5. ....
6. ....
7. ....
8. ....
9. ....
10. ....

Example
I am now more confident that I have more resources to assist me i.e. a better support group, this book and www.wellnessfitcoach.com website.

I can progress more confidently in the knowledge that I am well on my way to long-term weight loss success using the correct information and strategies.

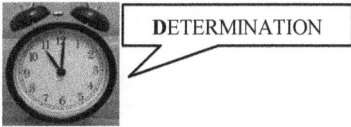

DETERMINATION

It's 11am. Self-determination is one of the most popular and widely tested approaches to motivation, and relates to the degree to which your behaviours are chosen and self-initiated. (AmPsych, 2000).

First of all you need to address whether you have any of the following:
- A lack of intention
- Feelings of incompetence
- Lack of connection between your behaviour and your dream goal
- Any external pressure i.e. weight loss is non-self-determined and not your idea
- You perceive weight loss to be mundane and not enjoyable.

Therefore:
- Identify your intention
- Increase your competence levels
- Connect your behaviour with your dream goal

137

- Reduce any external pressures i.e. ensure weight loss is self-determined and your idea
- Start to perceive weight loss as an ongoing life activity and make it enjoyable.

<u>Self-talk task</u>
These will all lead you onto your path to success. So how do we address these areas?

Write down at least 10 things related to determination that will assist you with this practice:

1. ....
2. ....
3. ....
4. ....
5. ....
6. ....
7. ....
8. ....
9. ....
10. ....

<u>Example</u>
Wanting to better my health because I want to be a role model to my children instead of a burden that I see myself as now, drives my self-determination. My determination is stronger than ever before because I want to be able to play with my children without getting out of breath, and I am determined to gain more energy by progressing with my food and exercise choices step-by-step.

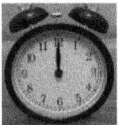

SELF-
ESTEEM

While body image and self-esteem are strongly linked, thinking you can solve all your problems by losing weight isn't realistic, and it may set you up for disappointment. (R.L. Duyff, 2006).

<u>Self-talk task</u>
It's 12 noon. Self-esteem related to weight loss. Write down at least 10 things related to esteem that will assist you with this practice:

1. ....
2. ....
3. ....
4. ....

5. ....
6. ....
7. ....
8. ....
9. ....
10. ....

<u>Example</u>
By asking myself specific questions such as: *What* is my dream goal? *Why* do I want to lose weight? How am I going to achieve my goals? The answer to such questions will increase my self-esteem substantially, and I will get my self-esteem to a level where I need it to be in order to be successful. I must also love all others and myself and have acceptance by allowing the people close to me to love and re-spect me in return.

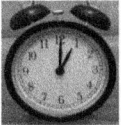

FOCUS

You do not have to define a goal weight. It is completely acceptable to begin your weight loss programme with the goal of losing an undefined amount of weight, fit-ting into a specific pair of clothes, or just becoming healthier and more active. Positive changes and clearly defined health-related goals may work just as well or even better. (M.B. Jampolis, 2007).

<u>Self-talk task</u>
It's 1pm. Focus related to weight loss. Write down at least 10 things related to focus that will assist you with this practice:
1. ....
2. ....
3. ....
4. ....
5. ....
6. ....
7. ....
8. ....
9. ....
10. ....

<u>Example</u>
In order to develop my confidence, my immediate focus is to commit to the follow-ing vision: to lose 2.2lbs or 1kg per week. These are small realistic steps and closer to my dream goal.

139

My focus assures me that my goals can be adjusted, as long as the reason is justified in order to optimise their potential effect on my life.

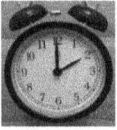

GRATITUDE

Studies have shown that being thankful can change the way you think or act. When you experience a sense of gratitude, you feel joyful, enlightened and uplifted. Gratitude is a very important part of the obtaining and maintaining your perfect weight. (K.F. Graham, 2007).

Self-talk task
It's 2pm. List down all the things you are grateful for on a daily basis. When you are grateful, all good things will happen around you because being grateful is one of the most important things in life. You can be grateful for everything you have, but some of the things we take for granted are sometimes the most important things i.e. for your health and the health of your family and close friends, running water, fresh bedding, to be able to see and smell flowers and hear the birds sing, etc.

Ideally, being grateful should be practiced first thing in the morning as you awake, and last thing at night before you go to sleep. Another good thing to do to prevent negative chatter at anytime is to repeat 'thank you' every step whilst walking, and even self-talk by saying what you are thankful for each or every other step.

Be grateful especially if you have one or more of the following:
- Love
- Family
- Health.

Write down at least 10 things related to gratitude that will assist you with this practice:
1. ....
2. ....
3. ....
4. ....
5. ....
6. ....
7. ....
8. ....
9. ....
10. ....

I am grateful for the health I have, the air that I breathe and the opportunities I have been blessed with in order to make the best use of my life. I realise that whatever issues I feel that I may have, that I must be grateful at all times because there is always someone in a worse situation than me.

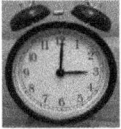

HAPPINESS

Happiness and well-being are the desired outcomes of positive psychology. (M.E.P. Seligman, 2002).

Self-talk task
It's 3pm. Happiness related to weight loss.Write down at least 10 things related to happiness that will assist you with this practice:

1. ....
2. ....
3. ....
4. ....
5. ....
6. ....
7. ....
8. ....
9. ....
10. ....

Example
I am happy that I get to wake up each and every day knowing that I have every chance to be one step closer to my dreams.

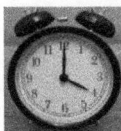

IMAGINATION

It's 4pm. Self-hypnosis is a method of inducing a deep state of relaxation and awareness, and related to weight loss you can aim to create simple mental images of your desired state i.e. *what you want?* You always maintain full control; therefore, it does not involve you having to go into a deep state of trance, and if you manage to effectively tap into the right side of your brain you can *improve your creativity* substantially (Percept & Motor Skills, 1996).

Write down at least 10 things related to imagination that will assist you with this practice:

1. ....
2. ....
3. ....
4. ....
5. ....
6. ....
7. ....
8. ....
9. ....
10. ....

Example
Using my imagination allows me to visualise and feel what it will be like to have exactly what I want. The more positive my thoughts are, the more chance I have of success and I can be safe in the knowledge that there is no limit to what I can imagine and visualise for myself.

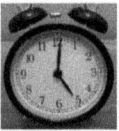

JUDGEMENT

If you have an internal judge (and who doesn't?) you may feel this type of internal division, which prevents you from loving yourself without judgment. But we can now change that, simply by taking the term 'love thyself' literally. (J. Good, 2003).

Self-talk task
It's 5pm. Judgement related to weight loss. Write down at least 10 things related to judgment that will assist you with this practice:

1. ....
2. ....
3. ....
4. ....
5. ....
6. ....
7. ....
8. ....
9. ....
10. ....

Example
My judgment should be tailored to what is right and what is going to get me what I

142

want. My judgment should hold me accountable to ensure I am making the correct choices in order for me to stay on the path to success. I must judge my decisions at all times, justifying that my nutrition and physical activity choices are keeping me on track.

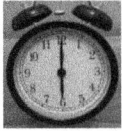

KNOWLEDGE

We live in a fast food world and our greatest nutrition enemy is rightly called JUNK. (L. Hammons, 2011).

Self-talk task
It's 6pm. Knowledge related to weight loss. Write down at least 10 things related to knowledge that will assist you with this practice:

1. ....
2. ....
3. ....
4. ....
5. ....
6. ....
7. ....
8. ....
9. ....
10. ....

Example
My knowledge is now on the correct path to success, and as I read this book the content ensures that I am up-to-date with what I have to do to reach my dreams quicker. My knowledge should of course be updated with the times and current trends, but only if the evidence has been researched and proven to be true. Wellness FitCoach allows me to visit their website as a lifelong member in order to access any information I am unsure of so that my knowledge is constantly updated.

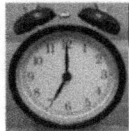

LONGEVITY

Permanent alterations in your lifelong attitudes toward diet and exercise are the keys to successful weight management. You must be motivated to change habits not for a few weeks or months, but for a lifetime. The importance of this must not be under-estimated. (J. Lawrence, L. Brown Wilder, S. Margolis & M.D. Cheskin, 2007).

It's 7pm. Longevity related to weight loss. Write down at least 10 things related to longevity that will assist you with this practice:

1. ....
2. ....
3. ....
4. ....
5. ....
6. ....
7. ....
8. ....
9. ....
10. ....

Example

My desire is to live through this era of poor health by changing something about the way I have lived my life so far. In simple terms and in order for me to live longer I need to get moving and eat healthier but in the correct manner as explained in this book and on the www.wellnessfitcoach.com website.

"To know the road ahead, ask those coming back"

- Chinese proverb

Smile and be happy

First and foremost your happiness is about appreciating what you already have by way of gratitude, also from being continuously aware of your thoughts, actions and your environment. Being thankful for what you already have in your life is a great start, although these types of things have already happened or are already in your life. What you need to attract is something that you want in the future 'before it occurs' so your imagination, your visualisation, your everyday thoughts should be grateful as if you already have it.

As Dr Joe Dispenza (2012) explains, 'you are moving:
* From *cause and effect*
* To *causing an effect* i.e. changing something inside of you to produce an effect outside of you.

The emotions as if it is a reality are very difficult to master, but he goes on to point out that your body which only understands feelings must be convinced that it has the emotional quotient of the future experience, happening to you now.

"Most folks are about as happy as they make up their minds to be."

- Abraham Lincoln (1809-1865)

144

Process goals

No more distractions
Nothing should stand in your way, no distractions and definitely no excuses, and if you set realistic process goals for yourself then you will achieve success every time. These can be daily or weekly goals, but 100% of your focus will be required without fail until each goal is met. It is very easy to become too critical when you focus on your outcome goal i.e. to lose 80kg, and this is understandable as it may seem a long way off. You must therefore, be realistic in the sense that you should at least know how long it has taken you to put on weight i.e. 5-10 years maybe? If you're honest with yourself it would more than likely have been a long process, but either way you must reduce the critical noise from within.

As Lynn Williams (2009) mentions; do what naturally motivated people do and focus on the benefits and the rewards, build in some feedback, enjoy your future and know how to troubleshoot.

Your new focus should be the processes you are going to undertake in order to get to where you want to get to. These process goals are achievable steps that you are going to take, but they must be realistic and agreed to by you prior to taking them. You should devote 100% of your focus and concentration on these small steps, and you should be engaged in the job at hand in order to get to the next phase whatever it takes.

♥Task 33
Lifestyle Challenge 4
Write down your outcome goal and the process goals in order to reach it. No matter how small your steps are you will get there in the end so long as you keep persevering.

Important
Prior to this you would have made yourself accountable and signed to say that you agree to the process goals that you have set yourself, purely because you know they are realistic and achievable. One thing is for sure, if you don't start you won't ever know, and if you continue to put things off you will always be wondering 'what if?'

Knowing that you are on the correct path to achieving what you want is enough reason to feel good about yourself. You are responsible for how happy you are, and when your positivity shines through you, this will ensure that you are capable of being happy all of the time. When you are doing everything you can possibly do to 'get it right' you will always be successful, no matter what.

- Get your thoughts right
- Eat well and exercise enough.

145

Your new thought process will automatically make you think better of yourself, your time will be better managed, and by utilising a more structured process of daily events, your success awaits.

The following list describes what you require for permanent weight loss success, and according to four psychology professors, (academic board) of The Mind Gym (2005), a few or all of the following factors are involved during your moments of greatest enjoyment:

1. You confront tasks that you have a chance of completing.

You now have in your possession this book so this will give you instant *confidence*.
2. You can concentrate on what you are doing.
Focus on completing your tasks and your step-by-step process goals.

3. You have clear goals.

Having *process goals* that are realistic and achievable will ensure you stay on track.

4. You have immediate feedback.

Feedback and *support* from not only your friends and family but from us too, also feedback from *how you feel* when you consume good nutrition and exercise wisely. According to Mihaly Csikszentmihaly (1997) our actions and feelings are always influenced by other people, whether they are present or not.

5. You have a deep and effortless involvement that is all embracing.

Involvement in the *tasks* and the *process goals* in order to keep you motivated.

6. You have a sense of control over your actions.

Read the book, complete the tasks and process goals, and set yourself new habits for a lifetime of success.

7. You don't think about yourself during the activity, but think better of your-self after you have completed it.

Think of this book as a project, a project that focuses only on Y.O.U and your families' health.

8. Your sense of the duration of time is altered.

Psychology, exercise & nutrition

Fear of failure and perfectionism are two of the main reasons why people procrastinate or avoid making decisions. In many ways putting off important daily tasks like 'exercise' and 'good nutrition' should not even come into your head, they should be as important as brushing your teeth or having a shower. However, you have to change the way you think because times have changed for the worst, and society is not allowing you to live as you should live.

Due to many factors life has been made far too easy for us, yet we are still expected to work hard, therefore constant day-to-day stress consequently leaves us limited time for ourselves. So you must regain control of your destiny and use your time more efficiently in order to be more relaxed but energised and involved with your day-to-day tasks.

- *Accept* that there's no such thing as a perfect human being
- *Trust* in your ability and do your best
- If it arises treat failure as *feedback* that you can learn from.

IMPORTANT
Your thoughts, daily exercise and eating healthily are the most important factors on your weight loss journey. So if for some reason you don't do your planned morning exercise then you need to do 30 minutes later that day, but you should try to not to get into exercise debt. Any exercise is better than none at all, so move away from the all or nothing way of thinking, take small steps (process goals) to change your habits. Remind yourself how motivated you feel when you have eaten well and exercised.

From your findings so far write down daily reminders about why you feel that nutrition and exercise are important to you and your desire to lose weight. For example, nutrition and exercise are important to me because without combining them I will find it very difficult to reach my goals; therefore, I must achieve my daily goals at all times.

7 steps to permanent weight loss success

1. Read the book from start to finish whilst attempting some of the tasks as you go - (♥ Tasks 1-33)

To avoid having high expectations and getting too overwhelmed with the tasks, just attempt the 'simplest actions' first i.e. only the actions you feel that you can implement into your life immediately. Then revisit the others until you have completed them all.

147

2. <u>Start and complete 21 days in a row, utilising everything you have learned in this book</u> (see guide below).

Once you have completed all the tasks, you have your goals and your plan of action, ensure your start date is set in concrete with no distractions. Be true to yourself by remaining fully accountable for your actions, and be positive at all times.

Your easy guide

3. Decide how you can make the appropriate 'mind/body' habitual changes - (♥Tasks 12, 23, 26, 27)

Realistic step-by-step changes
4. Choose which self-talk dialogue(s) you can implement effectively into your life (♥Task 12, pages 108, 120-122, 131-144)

The 'phrases' or 'affirmations' that you choose should really resonate with you, and these should ideally be in the future tense as if you already have what you want right now. The phrases you decide to use should summarise what you want the most of regarding your permanent weight loss success.

5. Ensure your daily choices (thoughts/nutrition/physical activity) are in line with your goals (page 128-131, 145-147)

For more permanent results choose more wisely and stay out of your comfort zone. Realistic process goals will take you progressively closer to your desired outcome.

6. Continue to take action and behave according to your values, beliefs and desires (♥Tasks 4, 5, 7, 15, 16)

If you change just a little something about the way you were before, you will definitely get different results.

7. Family-shopping-list (♥Tasks 2, 22 pages 53-60, 63-74)

Make the right choices irrespective of cost. Remember it's about fuelling yourself and your family for longevity not the short-term. There's more price to pay for an unhealthy and shorter life, so spend less time and money on something else not as important.

"Think 'health' and weight loss will follow."

– Wellness FitCoach

Part 7: ABOUT THE AUTHOR

What does the author do?

By way of an example, when you have a financial advisor trying to sell you something you should always ask 'what investments do you have? And so in this particular case we wanted to let you know what the author does. In brief I always *try* and do the following wherever I can:

Mind
- Always try and think before I speak
- As I am talking, try and think about what I am saying
- After I have spoken, try and analyse what I have said
- To always look on the bright side of life (cue for a song here)
- Look at everything as having happened for a reason
- Treat failure as feedback
- Turn negative thoughts into positive ones where possible.

Nutrition
- Try and always eat a variety of foods
- Hardly ever drink fizzy drinks
- Fast food as a treat and mostly limited to a takeaway at the weekend to take a break from cooking
- Eat masses of veggies in order to satisfy me and fill me up
- Try and cut back on my meat portions
- Try and eat more fruit
- Always in possession of a bottle of water (never leave home without one).

Physical activity
- Use a variety of methods to prevent boredom
- Swim once a week
- Run once a week
- Gym stuff 2-3 times a week depending on work routine.

Rest and meditation
I admit that I find it very difficult to get quiet time, but I am very good at listening to my body, so I know when it is time to relax and put my feet up. My justification in order to do this is down to what my day has been like i.e. have I achieved what I set out to do and has it been a productive day from a personal self-satisfying point of view? In short, most days I always try to do as much in the day as possible and use the time productively, and not waste a single second.

My meditation is different to most peoples and can occur unplanned and when I least expect it. That is to say that thoughts and visions come to me during the times when I am most relaxed. For example:

- Whilst driving (not advisable) – I always carry a pen in the car
- Whilst in the gym (always make notes during workouts)
- Always during cardio i.e. whilst swimming, running or recreational walking, etc. (very difficult to take notes LOL so rely on memory)
- Before sleeping and upon waking (pen and paper always by the bedside, hoping to remember dreams too).

Some of my life experiences

Self-achievement
- Royal Marines Commando - 8 month physically and mentally enduring course
- Receiving Green Beret
- Two Northern Ireland tours (rural & urban) – where I received a commendation, a highly-regarded award.

Self-doubt situations = (no 'time' for it)
1. Deploying to Norway – (Seven times) on arduous winter training missions. The first time I left home properly (for longer than a week) I still remember to this day calling my grandfather from Norway. I said I missed home and didn't really know if I could continue on, he replied very calm and collected and said, "At least you have a date where you know you will be coming home." I said "What do you mean?" He said, "Well in the war, we never knew when it would end, and IF we would come home at all." I had no answer for that and just got on with what I had to do to make the best of the situation I was in. From that moment on I accepted that no matter what you feel about your current situation, without doubt there will always be someone out there who has experienced what you have, and in most cases many people are worse off than you. My first Norway deployment made me doubt that I had made the correct career choice; I couldn't have been further from the truth.
2. Moving country – from the UK to the USA i.e. from the security of your own country. When doubt crept in all I did was look at 'what's the worse thing that can happen?' If it doesn't work and you return home then so be it. As it happened I looked at it as a large part of my life experience at the time. It always looks good on your CV that you have multicultural experience and the most important thing I learnt from it was that no matter how you weigh up the advantages/disadvantages, etc. One thing is for sure, 'Do not have any regrets in your life'. Make a decision based on positivity and ensure that you will not look back one day and say 'what if?' Remember – in life there is No failure…only feedback, so change any thoughts of doubt into a positive thought, into positive behaviours and then into positive actions!

Self-motivation

Pre-military training – RM – PTI. As a teenager, I was always motivated to be active in one way or another. Whether it was having one or more newspaper delivery rounds, working at the weekend as a silver service waiter or in a café as an assistant chef type, dishwashing run around. Then I started my first full-time job in a warehouse, and although this was only lifting boxes, it kept me active mentally and physically. But my true motivation came from talking to people who worked there. These were people I didn't know, I had nothing in common with them (apart from working in the same place), but they got to know me as I was their young run around; however, I was no pushover, so they were curious as to what made me tick. In a way I saw them as my guides for the future me.

At that stage of my life I was too young to have any kind of awareness of who I was and what I could become; therefore, I had no real ambition as such. Working there was an engineer for the large machinery, he was coming up to retirement and I just saw him as a very wise old man. In a nutshell he observed and listened to me and decided to invite me to a karate club, which was run by a former SAS friend of his. This visit got us talking about the military and martial arts, etc. but the main thing was to guide me onto bigger and better things instead of being cooped up in a warehouse/factory for the rest of my life.

Anyway, you all know the story of the 'law of attraction' and this particular era was the time of Bruce Lee films and Mike Tyson's climb to the top in the boxing world. In short, my direction had changed and my father decided it was time to take me to see if boxing was for me…and as it happened it was. My self-motivation drove me to go home after work and then go boxing for a few nights a week, which continued for a year or so. Then during one of my conversations with the wise old man at work, he mentioned why don't I join the military?

And so after many hours of grilling him into telling me about his career in the army I decided one day to go in my lunch break to the army and navy careers office. In the window I looked at the various posters and pictures, and one picture stood out for me more than the others, and that was the Royal Marines adverts. Pictures of skiing in Norway and patrolling in the Jungle of Brunei did it for me and got me motivated to get going. So I decided to go in and to cut a very long story short I had an interview, a medical and a 3-day selection. But then had to have a severe think about whether or not what I had experienced up until that moment was for me or not.

So, I went back to the old wise man and my grandfather who had served in the war with the army, to see if they could convince me. Whilst thinking, I upped the tempo and my new daily routine was as follows: run to the nearest swimming pool to my work, swim for ½ an hr., then run to work, do a full days work and then run to the boxing club, train for 1-2 hours then run home. My motivation even went as far as running and swimming in old army issue clothing that I had purchased from a local store – boots n' all. Not forgetting filling a rucksack with house bricks till I could fit

151

no more in and plodding around for miles and miles with that on my back, amongst other crazy things!

Although there are many other examples for how fine-tuned my self-motivation is, my point ends by sharing with you a comment made by my instructor on my Royal Marine PTI course, he said, "Today you are the fittest you will ever be" and the first thing that came into my mind was disagreement. Not because we weren't fit, of course we were. We had the best training in the world and then to be trained by the elite of the military fitness world, of course we were fit. My disagreement was purely because my belief is that my desire, in this case to be a Royal Marine Physical Training Instructor *originated* from my self-motivation and then my continued self-perseverance, which kept me going i.e. all from within. Not from being motivated from an outside source i.e. a personal trainer or military instructor.

Being the fittest or best at what you do, this is kind of an end product, also being spurred on by supporters to get a better time on a run will get you to your peak. But it's your self-motivation that gets you there in the first place, this is your inner strength and from your self-motivation.

Having faith, belief and not giving up
On one occasion when I was injured, physically delirious and had no map, I managed to reach my objective to pass a demanding selection course. Because I had no map, I used the ground I'd previously covered, the stars and specific reference points to steer me. This was one of those times I asked my 'internal guide' for help. Whatever your thoughts are on that doesn't really matter, as it worked for me then and has done since on a few other occasions too.

Self-talk
When you prepare yourself mentally, you can be rest assured that you will be ready for almost anything. *Every day* during my 6-month tour in Northern Ireland, I prepared myself fully for any eventuality i.e. what I would say on the military radio and exactly what I would do. One night, four months into the tour, I was shining my torch behind some railings and came across an explosive device that was hidden from view from the main road. I immediately took action and dealt with the incident with ease, as my pre-recorded action plan was so well rehearsed that everything fell into place. The ops room were dumbfounded to hear my radio communication – most people in those situations freeze and panic. The point to note here is that with sound planning and preparation, daily self-talk and confidence, you can deal with any given situation.

Self-discipline
RM Physical Training Instructor – 16-weeks of arduous training, from learning basic medical topics to learning how to coach, mentor and get the average civilian (potential RM) physically fit. Once qualified, then trained 100's of men to become Britain's elite.

<u>Rehabilitation Therapist</u> – Studied on a 9-month full-time course learning clinical anatomy, kinesiology, exercise therapy, anatomy and physiology. Upon graduation fixed the Marines when sick or injured through motivation and specific rehabilitation plans.

Post UK Military

Left the UK to become Director of Fitness for a brand new fitness facility in the USA. Set the centre up from scratch and turned it into a major contender within the surrounding states.

Other International Work

Recently and for almost 11 years now, I have been working for the UAE government, advising top military commanders on all Health and Fitness issues in an extremely high profile role. I can speak, read and write in the Arabic language.

Specific Qualifications

The qualifications I am most proud of are a degree level course with the American College of Sports Medicine (ACSM), at which I studied whilst working full-time to achieve the Health Fitness Specialist qualification (HFS). I also travelled to Miami, where I completed a Neuro-Linguistic Programming (NLP) practiitioners course that helped me deal with some of my own personal demons and past issues. I have always wanted a degree but I decided that I could pursue this route later in life, as I will not always be able to travel. So after leaving the UK military, travelling to the US (instead of achieving higher education) was a tough decision for me.

In addition to the above, as well as being an ex-royal marine commando physical training instructor/remedial specialist, my best achievement so far (apart from meeting my wife and starting a family) was when I was accepted into the MSC Sport and Exercise Psychology programme based on my current qualifications, life experience and commitment within the health and fitness industry (without actually having an undergraduate degree).

Sporting Career

A participant in all major sporting events but mainly in boxing. I am also an ABA coach, a keen skier and snowboarder as well as a skiing instructor/teacher.

Fitness Achievements

I have completed two marathons, won individual and group fitness competitions as well as winning all my boxing fights.

Other Work Committments

I teach, assess and internally verify for specific health and fitness courses for some of the most recognised international awarding bodies. Alongside the day-to-day management of the WellnessFit Coach website for weight loss clients, I also undertake V.I.P personal training from time to time, although only for recommended or referred clients. I offer courses for those wanting to get into the fitness industry, and those already qualified who want to continue their professional development. I've written a number of books related to helping people get the best from themselves and I assist a few charities via various means.

153

Part 8: REFERENCES

AmPsych (2000). 55, 68-78. 140

Astrup, A., Grunwald, G.K., Melanson, E.L., Saris, W.H.M., & Hill, J.O. (2000). "The Role of Low-Fat Diets in Body Weight Control: A Meta-analysis of Ad Libitum Dietary Intervention Studies." *International Journal of Obesity, 24,* 1545-1552. 48

Baumeister, R. F., & Tierney, J., (2011). *Willpower - rediscovering the greatest human strength, USA,* Penguin group (USA) (pp.215-219). 108

Beck, J., *Cognitive Therapy for Weight Loss.*   30

Biddle, S. J. H., & Mutrie, N., (2008). *Psychology of physical activity.* Oxon, UK Routledge (p.354). 104

Boyes, C., (2006). *Need to know?* NLP. London, UK, Collins. (pp.14, 18-21). 4, 9, 33,

Brookes, D., (1999). Your Personal Trainer, (p.49). IL, USA. Human kinetics. 85

Brooks, E. R., (2010). *Choose happiness now, your positive action plan for a life of happiness,* (p.22). Los Angeles: Evelyn Brooks. 137

Cummins Dr. D., June 21, 2013. *How to boost your willpower.* http://m.psychologytoday.com/blog/good-thinking/201306/how-boost-your-willpower). 108

Csikszentmihaly, M., (1997). *Finding flow - the psychology of engagement with everyday life,* N.Y, USA. Basic books, (pp.12-13.) 123,150

Dispenza, J., (2012). *Breaking the habit of being yourself.* London, UK. Hay House UK Ltd. (p.26). 148

Duyff, R. L., (2006). *American Dietetic association complete food and nutrition guide,* (3rd ed.). New Jersey: John Wiley and sons. 142

Ellis, A., (1953). *Rational Emotive Behaviour Therapy (REBT). Behaviour therapies of a cognitive nature.* 31

Ello-Martin, J.A., (2005). 63

Elwood, et al., *British Heart Journal, 69,* 183-187. 81

Engler, B., (2009). *Personality theories* (8th ed.). 20 Boston, USA. Houghton Mifflin Harcourt publishing company. (p.251). 35

Gallup, R., *The G.I. (Glycemic Index) Diet.* 60

Geller, J., Cockell, S.J., Hewitt, P.L., Goldner, E.M. & Flett G.L., (2000). Department of Psychiatry, University of British Columbia, Vancouver, British Columbia. *Int J Eat Disorde*r, 28(1) 8-19. 19

Good, J., (2003). *Weight loss: How to keep your commitment.* (p.71). Oregon: Wet Cat eBooks. 146

Graham, K.F., (2007). *Perfect weight: the secret to weight loss and keeping it off.* (1st ed.) Atlanta, Ga: Success in U LLC. (p.261).143

Gross, R. D., (1992). *Psychology, the science of mind and behaviour,* (2nd ed.). London, UK. Hodder and Stoughton. (p.811). 43

Grotto, D., (2007). *101 foods that could save your life.* NY, USA bantam books. (pp.10, 18, 19, 47, 61, 71, 128, 138, 155, 159, 194, 206, 217, 237, 270, 274, 281, 315, 325, 347, 350). 60

Hammons, L., (2011). *Knowledge is lonely: if it isn't shared,* (p.171), Indianapolis, USA: Xlibris corporation. 146

Hellenic, J., Psych (2006). *3,* 164-175. 140

Holford, P., (2006). *The low-GL diet made easy.* London, UK. Little brown book group. (pp.30,31, 40, 42). 46, 54

I Journal of Obesity, (1994). *18,* 145-154. 53.

Jampolis, M.B., (2007). *The busy persons guide to permanent weight loss.* Tennessee: Thomas Nelson, Inc. 142

Jones, D.C., (2004). University of Washington, Thorbjorg Helga Vigfusdottir, Reykjavik University, Yoonsun Lee, University of Washington. *"Body dissatisfaction and psychological factors, Journal of Developmental Psychology.* 19

Lawrence. J., Brown Wilder, L., Margolis, S. & Cheskin, M.D., (2007). *Nutrition and weight control for longevity.* (p.59). Bethel, CT: Medletter Associates LLC. 147

Liao, K.L., (2000). 29

Litvinoff, S., (2004). *The confidence plan.* London, UK, BBC books. (pp.186-189). 110

McCullagh, P., PhD., Stiehl, J., & Weiss, W.R., (1990). *"Developmental modelling effects on the quantitative and qualitative aspects of motor performance."* 77

Medicine and science in sports and exercise, (1994) 26(5), supplement, (p.559). 50

Mood and human performance: Conceptual, Measurement, and Applied issues. (2006). Nova Science Publishers (pp.1-35). 104

Neil, K., & Holford, P., (1998). *Balancing hormones naturally.* (p.30, 161)London, UK. Judy Piatkus publishers Ltd. 26

Paul, G. (2009). *Perfect detox.* (p.22). London, UK. Random house books. 50

Paxton, S. J., Neumark-Sztainer, D., Hannan, P. J., Eisenberg, M., (2006). Body dissatisfaction prospectively predicts depressive symptoms and low self-esteem in adolescent girls and boys. *Journal of Clinical Child and Adolescent Psychology, 35*, 539-549. *19*

Percept & Motor Skills, (1996). *83*, 1347-1352. 145

Price, R, A., (2008). *Glycemic Matrix Guide to Low GI and GL Eating*, (p.19). West Conshohocken, PA. Infinity publishing. 57

Seligman, M.E.P., (2002). *Authentic happiness: using the new positive psychology to realise your potential for lasting fulfilment. (*p.261). New York: Simon & Shuster. 144

Starks, T.P., (2006). *Focus on nutrition research.* (p.92). New York: Nova science publishers, Inc. 139

Stipek, (1996). *The Oxford Handbook of Human Motivation, 2012.* (p.467). Oxford university press Inc., New York, USA. 80

The Mind Gym, (2005). (pp.205-214) Time Warner book group, London, UK. 109,149

University of Sydney/
http://lowcarbdiets.about.com/od/whattoeat/a/glycemicindlist.htm
Gallup, R., *The G.I. (Glycemic Index) Diet.* 59

Vale, J., (2012). *The juice master diet.* (pp.216-222). London, UK, Harper Collins. 71

Waller, D. L., (2011). *Sustainable weight loss, the definitive guide to a healthy body weight.* (p183). Bloomington, IN: iUniverse. 138
Whitten, H., (2009). *Cognitive behavioural coaching techniques.* (p.355). Sussex, UK. John Wiley and sons Ltd. 25

Williams, L., (2009). *Perfect positive thinking.* (pp.35-51). London, UK. Random House books. 112,148

Young, Dr. R.O. & Young, S., (2002). *PH Miracle, reclaim your health.* NY, USA. Warner books Inc. (pp.155-). 45

Useful websites:

www.awlr.org

www.athealth.com/Consumer/disorders/Bingeeating.html

www.arthritistoday.org

www.bestdietforme.com

http://www.dailymail.co.uk/health/article-1195904/Is-healthy-brown-loaf-just-white-bread-dyed.html

http://www.diabetes.org.uk/Guide-to-diabetes/Food_and_recipes/The-Glycaemic-Index/

http://www.doctoroz.com

www.drfuhrman.com

http://www.drweil.com/drw/u/PAG00361/anti-inflammatory-food-pyramid.html

EzineArticles.com/119399

www.foodrevolution.org

www.humankinetics.com

www.lifestylewtloss.com

http://lowcarbdiets.about.com/od/whattoeat/a/glycemicindlist.htm

www.mayoclinic.com

www.medicalnewstoday

www.nhlbi.nih.gov

www.optimumbodysculpting.com

www.paulamee.com/paulamee/Main/Eating_Well_GI_Guide.htm

www.pponline.co.uk/ency/goal-setting.html

www.resolutions.bz

www.selfgrowth.com

http://www.theenergytherapycentre.co.uk/eft-explained.htm

www.web4health.info

http://www.webmd.com/diet/your-omega-3

www.weight-dieting.org

www.weightlosspsychology.com

www.wellnessfitcoach.com

http://lowcarbdiets.about.com/od/whattoeat/a/glycemicindlist.htm

http://www.wholefoodsmarket.com/healthy-eating/health-starts-here/resources-and-tools/top-ten-andi-scores

www.wikipedia.com

INDEX